DISPATCHES FROM THE LAND OF ALZHEIMER'S

Daniel Gibbs is a retired n[...], with early-stage Alzheimer's [...]. Having spent [...] years caring for patients, many with dementia themselves, he is now an active advocate for the early recognition and management of Alzheimer's. He has written previously about his experiences as seen from two points of view, doctor and patient, in *A Tattoo on my Brain: A Neurologist's Personal Battle against Alzheimer's Disease* (Cambridge University Press, 2021 and 2023 [revised edition]).

"Dr. Daniel Gibbs taught me neurology when I was in training, and he continues to teach me thirty years later. In *A Tattoo on my Brain* and in his speaking and advocacy, he turned the bad luck of his Alzheimer's disease into gifts for the rest of us: rare insights, thoughtful analysis, and an inspiring example of how to live and thrive in the face of great challenges. *Dispatches from the Land of Alzheimer's* is his latest gift, weaving together personal experiences, reasoned commentary on "pop science", analysis of cutting-edge research, good advice on a brain-healthy lifestyle, and through it all the reminder to "live in the moment".

Joseph Quinn, MD, FAAN Ericksen Endowed Professor for Neurodegeneration Research, Parkinson's Center Director, Department of Neurology, Oregon Health and Science University

"Daniel Gibbs is a warrior. And that's a blessing to him and to the world!

We are members of a club that neither of us wanted to join. I met Daniel over the phone a few years ago; we both had been diagnosed with Alzheimer's. I encouraged Daniel to write about this serpentine journey, as I have done. Over time, Daniel has inspired me to make lemonade without the lemons – the bittersweet of life. Those on this trek are best to write and talk about it, to tell their own stories, as Daniel has done as a neurologist who has been on both sides of this aisle; first as a doctor, now as a patient. As scripture notes in Luke 4:23, "Physician, heal thyself." The only conundrum is Daniel cannot – the plight of millions diagnosed with Alzheimer's and other dementias, as the experts race for a cure. Dispatches from the Land of Alzheimer's delivers in all ways as a soulful, edifying roadmap into this prowling demon of a disease."

Greg O'Brien, author, On Pluto: Inside the Mind of Alzheimer's

"What is it like to be a person living with Alzheimer's disease? In his collection of essays, Dispatches from the Land of Alzheimer's, Dan Gibbs provides a detailed, clear, vivid and candid account. Detailed and clear because he's a retired neurologist with a keen understanding of science. Vivid and candid because he's a person living with the disease. These poignant essays recount his experiences with loss of smell, changes in empathy, face blindness, making sense of the biomarkers of the disease as they misfold in his own brain, and day-to-day challenges like carrying on a conversation and working. Dan Gibbs has a notable talent to feel both sides of an experience – the losses and the gains. This book ought to be required reading for anyone who wants to live well with Alzheimer's disease."

Jason Karlawish, author of The Problem of Alzheimer's: How Science, Culture, and Politics Turned a Rare Disease into a Crisis and What We Can Do About It

"Dr. Gibbs' book is an honest, upbeat, moving and informative story of his journey through an Alzheimer's diagnosis and its aftermath. His indomitable spirit permeates every page."

Professor Adriane Fugh-Berman, Director, PharmedOut, Georgetown University Medical Center.

Dispatches from the Land of Alzheimer's

DANIEL GIBBS
Emeritus of Oregon Health and Science University

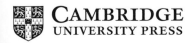

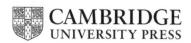

Shaftesbury Road, Cambridge CB2 8EA, United Kingdom

One Liberty Plaza, 20th Floor, New York, NY 10006, USA

477 Williamstown Road, Port Melbourne, VIC 3207, Australia

314–321, 3rd Floor, Plot 3, Splendor Forum, Jasola District Centre,
New Delhi – 110025, India

103 Penang Road, #05–06/07, Visioncrest Commercial, Singapore 238467

Cambridge University Press is part of Cambridge University Press & Assessment,
a department of the University of Cambridge.

We share the University's mission to contribute to society through the pursuit of
education, learning and research at the highest international levels of excellence.

www.cambridge.org
Information on this title: www.cambridge.org/9781009430050

DOI: 10.1017/9781009430067

First published 2024

Printed in the United Kingdom by TJ Books Limited, Padstow Cornwall

A catalogue record for this publication is available from the British Library.

Library of Congress Cataloging-in-Publication Data
Names: Gibbs, Daniel, author.
Title: Dispatches from the land of Alzheimer's / Daniel Gibbs.
Description: Cambridge, United Kingdom ; New York, NY, USA : Cambridge University Press,
2023. | Includes bibliographical references and index.
Identifiers: LCCN 2023031195 (print) | LCCN 2023031196 (ebook) | ISBN 9781009430050
(paperback) | ISBN 9781009430067 (epub)
Subjects: MESH: Alzheimer Disease | Neurologists | Oregon | Personal Narrative |
Collected Work
Classification: LCC RC523 (print) | LCC RC523 (ebook) | NLM WT 7 |
DDC 616.8/311–dc23/eng/20230828
LC record available at https://lccn.loc.gov/2023031195
LC ebook record available at https://lccn.loc.gov/2023031196

ISBN 978-1-009-43005-0 Paperback

[Medical disclaimer:]

Dedicated to the memory of my parents,
Zack Edward Gibbs and Elizabeth Martin Gibbs

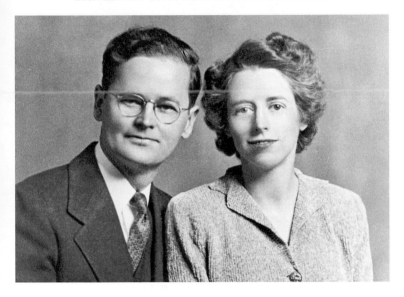

LOST IN THOUGHT

What was that plan I made in the shower?
It slipped down the drain just out of my grasp,
Long gone by the time I toweled dry.

What was that story on the radio today?
I know it was good and I'm trying to remember.
Maybe I'll recall if I drive by the place where I heard it.

What are the names of the neighbors next-door?
They've lived there for years, but I just can't remember.
Their names might return in a flash, in a minute,
    A few hours,
        A few days ….

I stand around lost in thought
But too often the thought is lost.

Damn, what was I thinking?

November 23, 2013

CONTENTS

Color plates can be found between pages 84 and 85

Unless otherwise noted, all photographs were either taken by the author or are from his personal collection.

ACKNOWLEDGMENTS

Thank you to Anna Whiting and her team at Cambridge University Press for believing in this book from the start and marshaling it through the editing and production process at what seemed at times to be warp speed. Thanks to Dr. Gil Rabinovici at the University of California, San Francisco, for allowing me to use the PET scans of my brain. Dr. Joseph Quinn at Oregon Health and Science University has been a friend and colleague for many years, and more recently, he has been my neurologist and guide as I enter the dementia phase of Alzheimer's disease. Thanks for being there, Joe.

Cambridge University Press and I are grateful to the publications that have kindly allowed for us to adapt articles originally published within their pages: *Alzheimer's Today* (the official publication of The Alzheimer's Foundation of America),[1] *Ageing Research Reviews*, and *Scientific American*.

A special thank you to my wife of 50 years, Lois Seed. With the sharp eyes of a retired librarian, Lois was the first, second, and third reader of this book. She encouraged me to add more personal anecdotes, and she called me to task when my writing became potentially inaccessible to lay readers. Thank you for everything Lois.

---

[1] The Alzheimer's Foundation of America is a nonprofit organization whose mission is to provide support, services, and education to individuals, families, and caregivers affected by Alzheimer's disease and related dementias nationwide and to fund research for better treatment and a cure. Its services include a National Toll-Free Helpline (866-232-8484) staffed by licensed social workers, the National Memory Screening Program, educational conferences and materials, and the "AFA Partners in Care" dementia care training for healthcare professionals. For more information about AFA, call 866-232-8484 or visit www.alzfdn.org. AFA holds the Charity Navigator's top four-star rating for its commitment to fiscal efficiency, transparency, and accountability.

PROLOGUE

Recently, I spoke to a group of medical students about Alzheimer's disease. I have been giving these talks three or four times a year for the last five years now. I know a lot about Alzheimer's disease because I am a retired neurologist, and I have treated many patients with dementia, including Alzheimer's disease.

I also know a lot because now I *have* mild Alzheimer's dementia. As we'll see in Chapter 3, Alzheimer's dementia is the late stage of Alzheimer's disease when cognitive impairment interferes with activities of daily living. The pathological changes in the brain caused by Alzheimer's disease begin to appear up to 20 years before the onset of cognitive impairment.

In retrospect, my first symptom of Alzheimer's disease occurred in 2006 when I was 55 and realized that my sense of smell was not as sharp as it once had been. I assumed it was due to normal aging. I wasn't particularly worried until, while doing genealogical research in 2012, I unexpectedly discovered that I have two copies of the *APOE*-4 allele, putting me at very high genetic risk for dementia later in life. Alzheimer's disease had not been on my radar screen because both my parents had died in midlife from cancer. I had taken care of many patients with dementia as a neurologist, but most of these, especially early in my career, had been in the late stages of the disease. I retired in 2013 at age 62 even though I did not yet have any measurable cognitive impairment.

Two years later, I volunteered for my first research study, an investigation of a then new positron emission tomography (PET) scan that could detect the abnormal tau protein in the neurofibrillary tangles of Alzheimer's. During this study, I had beta-amyloid and tau PET scans, an MRI scan, and two days of cognitive testing. The results showed that I had mild cognitive impairment (MCI) primarily affecting verbal memory, a moderate amount of beta-amyloid throughout my brain, and the beginnings of abnormal tau in my medial temporal lobes where it first appears in most cases of Alzheimer's disease. When the studies were repeated in 2018 and again in 2022, the cognitive tests were a little worse and the abnormal amyloid and tau had spread further throughout my brain. By 2022, I had mild Alzheimer's dementia.

It is important to realize that although I had significant amounts of Alzheimer's pathology in my brain in 2015, I was still doing pretty well cognitively although not well enough to continue working as a neurologist. I was still reading over 100 books per year. I could still balance the checkbook. I did have increasing problems with remembering names and coming up with the right words to say, but I got around some of these problems by using mnemonics. I volunteered for another study, the phase 3 trial of the anti-amyloid monoclonal antibody, aducanumab. Unfortunately, I had severe side effects of brain swelling and bleeding after just four doses, resulting in two days of intensive care unit (ICU) management and a slow recovery over the next few months [1]. These side effects are called amyloid related imaging abnormalities (ARIA). They were common in the study, occurring in over 40% of participants, but most of the time they were very mild and often asymptomatic. I was among only 2% who suffered severe ARIA requiring hospitalization, but I fully recovered with no persistent damage, except for the residual blood pigments left in my brain called hemosiderin. I call this the "tattoo on my brain" because the hemosiderin still shows up as black dots on my MRI scans. This actually was the inspiration for me to start writing about my experiences with Alzheimer's, which resulted in my first book: *A Tattoo on my Brain: A Neurologist's Personal Battle against Alzheimer's Disease*. I began with an opinion paper directed at other neurologists urging early recognition and management of Alzheimer's [2]. I then expanded that into a book for lay readers [3] that explains how it is possible to decrease the risk for and slow the progression of the disease through lifestyle modifications, especially when started early. I am hopeful that new drugs will prove effective at slowing or even stopping the progression of Alzheimer's, but I suspect that they will need to be used early in the disease, perhaps even before the start of cognitive impairment.

My Alzheimer's disease is progressing slowly. Now, in the spring of 2023, my reading speed has clearly decreased, primarily because I often have to go back and reread the previous page. I won't make 100 books this year. I'll probably be lucky to read 80. I can no longer balance the checkbook, and my wife, Lois, has taken over management of the household finances and planning. I have increasing trouble understanding other people when they speak, especially in a group. But I am still writing emails almost every day. With email, as opposed to live conversation, I have all the time I need to craft a sentence and figure out what I am trying to say. On the other hand, in-person communication is getting steadily worse. My ability to understand the spoken word is rapidly deteriorating. Some of this may be due to poor hearing, but most of the problem comes from the inability to understand what people are saying. I particularly have trouble when there are several people involved in the conversation, or worse, multiple simultaneous conversations. I can't untangle the words. My verbal output is also getting worse. I frequently use the wrong words, especially if I'm feeling stressed. It may be humorous in a family setting, but it is embarrassing in public.

It should be no surprise that people with Alzheimer's disease can still write. Perhaps the best examples are in the wonderful memoirs of Thomas DeBaggio, *Losing My Mind: An Intimate Look at Life with Alzheimer's*, and Greg O'Brien, *On Pluto: Inside the Mind of Alzheimer's*. Verbal memory is affected early in most people with Alzheimer's. That makes retrieving the right word at the right time difficult, particularly during speech. But writing seems to make word retrieval easier for me. I think this is because it provides an immediate link to the thoughts that have just come before. I can literally look back on the page to remind myself what I am trying to say. By contrast, when I am being interviewed or speaking without notes, I almost always lose the thread of what I am trying to communicate. I enjoy writing, and I think it keeps my mind sharper.

This book is a collection of essays I have written over the last few years. While this writing has been therapeutic for me, perhaps preserving some neuronal connections in my brain, my hope in sharing these essays is that others will learn something useful for their own personal journeys.

References

1   VandeVrede L, Gibbs DM, Koestler M, *et al.* Symptomatic amyloid-related imaging abnormalities in an ApoE-ε4/ε4 patient treated with aducanumab. *Alzheimers Dement: DADM* 2020; 12: e12101. https://doi.org/10.1002/dad2.12101 (open access).

2   Gibbs, DM. Early awareness of Alzheimer disease: A neurologist's personal perspective. *JAMA Neurology* 2019; 76: 249. https://doi.org/10.1001/jamaneurol.2018.4910.

3   Gibbs D, Barker TH. *A Tattoo on my Brain: A Neurologist's Personal Battle against Alzheimer's Disease,* (second edition). Cambridge: Cambridge University Press, 2023.

1 PHYSICIAN HEAL THYSELF

An email with a black box warning! That's what I got 11 years ago after Lois and I submitted saliva samples to a DNA testing service. Lois is the family genealogist, and she thought that DNA testing would be helpful in filling in some of the missing branches of our ancestral trees. In addition to lists of DNA relatives, the report included many risk genes for a variety of medical conditions, none of which were present for either of us. However, this locked black box contained two genes of neurological interest. A mutation in the *LRRK-2* gene is the most common cause of hereditary Parkinson's disease, and the *APOE-4* allele is the most significant genetic risk factor for late-onset Alzheimer's disease.

I am a general neurologist, and I knew about these neurological risk genes. About six years before this, I had started to lose my sense of smell. I thought this was most likely due to normal aging, but within five years I could not smell anything. I also had illusory odors, called phantosmias. These were like the smell of baking bread mixed with perfume. At first, these smells occurred several times a week and lasted a few minutes. Over the next few years, they became less frequent and finally disappeared entirely. About 80% of people with Parkinson's disease lose their sense of smell, usually some years before the tremor and gait problems develop. Phantosmias have been reported in people with Parkinson's disease. Given my olfactory symptoms, I wondered if I might be on the path to Parkinson's disease, so I unlocked the black box to see if

I had the *LRRK-2* mutation. I didn't have that. What I did have was two copies of the *APOE-4* allele giving me a 50% chance of having a diagnosis of Alzheimer's dementia by the age of 70 and making it almost certain that I would have it by the age of 80. It turns out that virtually all people with Alzheimer's disease have at least some loss of smell, but most are not aware of it until tested. My loss of smell had been my canary in the coal mine, but I had been unaware of its significance. Before getting my *APOE-4* results, Alzheimer's was just not on my radar screen. Both of my parents had died in midlife from cancer, but looking back a generation or two, there clearly was a family history of dementia.

I was stunned by this news. I was 61 years old and still active, teaching neurology to residents and medical students, and providing care for a variety of patients with neurological problems, including dementia. I traveled to Tanzania every year to teach neurology there as well. Cognitively, I thought I was still doing fine, but I asked a friend who is a dementia specialist to do some cognitive testing on me. Everything was normal, but there were some caveats. In all cognitive domains but one I scored in the 95th percentile. However, in verbal memory, I was in the 50th percentile, still normal, but it was a sign that there might already be some subtle damage to the part of my brain that deals with language.

A year later, when I was 62, I retired. I wanted to make sure that I didn't wait until I made a mistake in the care of my patients. I plunged into the neurological literature to find out what was known about slowing the progression of Alzheimer's disease. I found that there was consistent evidence that regular aerobic exercise can slow progression of the disease by as much as 50%. Plant-based diets such as the Mediterranean diet or a variant called the Mediterranean-DASH Intervention for Neurodegenerative Delay (MIND) diet with a greater emphasis on berries and nuts have been shown to slow progression by 30–50%. Other lifestyle modifications that appear to be beneficial include staying intellectually and socially active, getting at least seven hours of sleep per night, and controlling cardiovascular risk factors such as diabetes, high blood pressure, increased cholesterol, obesity, and smoking. Fortunately, I quit smoking when I was 18, and I follow these other guidelines religiously. I think it is making a difference.

I also want to do everything I can to help move the science about Alzheimer's forward. I have participated in six research studies so far. These include three clinical trials of medications, two technology-based studies, and a longitudinal neuroimaging study using amyloid and tau PET scans to follow the progression of Alzheimer's in my brain. I don't expect that any of these studies will cure me, but I hope that, by my participation, we can come a little bit closer to finding solutions to prevent, slow, or even reverse this disease.

I feel strongly that people with Alzheimer's disease and their families should feel comfortable talking about their journeys with family members, friends, and neighbors, and, if possible, with the general public. Stigma and misconceptions must be addressed. For example, the pathological changes in the brain, the amyloid plaques and tau-containing neurofibrillary tangles, appear very early, as much as 20 years before any cognitive issues arise. These 20 years before cognitive decline begins may well turn out to be the most effective time to stop or at least slow disease progression. Several current studies are looking at the efficacy of treatment in this presymptomatic period. But overcoming the stigma of Alzheimer's can be a barrier to recruiting research subjects who are at risk but who do not yet have cognitive impairment.

Although I was uneasy at first, I have come to enjoy talking to people about Alzheimer's disease. I have written a book about my experiences for the general public titled

A Tattoo on my Brain: A Neurologist's Personal Battle against Alzheimer's Disease, and I have given over 35 interviews and talks for radio, television, podcasts, newspapers, magazines, medical students, book groups, and Alzheimer support groups.

My Alzheimer's disease is slowly progressing. My most recent cognitive tests put me at the border between MCI and early Alzheimer's dementia. There is more amyloid and tau on my recent PET scans. But I am adapting to changes with the support of my wife, family, and friends. Life is still good, and I expect it to continue being good for many years to come.

Note: This essay is based on an article with a similar title published in Alzheimer's TODAY: The Official Magazine of the Alzheimer's Foundation of America, 2023; Volume 18, Number 1, pp. 18–19; a quarterly publication of the Alzheimer's Foundation of America https://alzfdn.org/wp-content/uploads/2023/03/ALZ-TODAY-18.1_MECH-HR.pdf.

2 EVALUATING NEW ADVANCES IN ALZHEIMER'S RESEARCH
Separating Hype from Fact

We all know that Alzheimer's is an enormous problem. Thousands of researchers around the world are tirelessly searching for clues that might lead to a solution – how to slow or prevent Alzheimer's. Reports of new findings are in the news almost daily. How do we know what is potentially important?

Science progresses a little like the building of a pyramid. The blocks of the pyramid are hypotheses, informed guesses about how something might work. A hypothesis is tested in an experiment. If proven true, the hypothesis becomes a block in the pyramid supporting and informing the next layer. If false, it is modified and retested or discarded. Block by block, layer by layer, the pyramid grows until ultimately the last block is laid at the top, and a theory is accepted, at least for the present. Unlike building a pyramid, science is fluid. Previous theories that had seemed sound may be challenged by new discoveries leading to reevaluation of the theory. The pyramid may need some modification.

Evaluating the potential importance of new discoveries depends on the collective assessment by other scientists working in the field. This results in a peer-reviewed paper in a medical or scientific journal. For papers submitted to

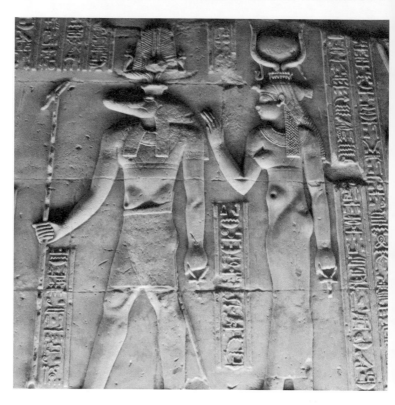

Temple of Edfu, Upper Egypt.

top journals such as *The New England Journal of Medicine*, *JAMA*, *BMJ*, *Science*, *Nature*, *The Lancet*, and many others, this vetting is very rigorous, and the majority of papers submitted may be rejected. Lay publications vary in the rigor with which they report on new discoveries. There are a number of news outlets with good science reporters – among my favorites and most trusted are *The New York Times* and *The Washington Post*. All of their science and medical writers are excellent, and several experts in the field are almost always consulted for articles about new advances. For those wanting to delve more deeply into the science behind recent advances in Alzheimer's research, I recommend *Alzforum*, a website for discourse among Alzheimer's experts [1]. Every Monday morning at 7 am Pacific time, I check the website for the weekly discussion of recent important papers. An accessible overview of our current knowledge of Alzheimer's disease is the Alzheimer's Association's 128-page *2023 Alzheimer's Disease Facts and Figures*, an authoritative monograph for general readers that is updated annually [2]. On the other extreme are stories originating from pharmaceutical company press releases before any publication in a peer-reviewed journal. Take these with a grain of salt.

Books about Alzheimer's disease may be harder to evaluate for accuracy. If published by an academic press, these books will have been reviewed by academic peers just like a scientific paper. Blogs, including my own [3], and most other social media posts generally have no outside review, no fact-checking at all, so *caveat emptor*!

References

1   *Alzforum – Networking for a Cure*. www.alzforum.org.
2   *2023 Alzheimer's Disease Facts and Figures*. www.alz.org/media/documents/alzheimers-facts-and-figures.pdf.
3   Gibbs D. *A Tattoo on my Brain*. https://tattooonmybrain.com.

3 ALZHEIMER'S DEMENTIA OR ALZHEIMER'S DISEASE

What's the Difference and Why Should We Care?

I now have a special interest in Alzheimer's disease. For nearly 25 years, I practiced general neurology in Portland, Oregon. Some of my patients had dementia, a progressive neurological disorder that causes severe cognitive impairment affecting memory, language, motivation, and mood, interfering with everyday activities. There are several diseases that can cause dementia, including Lewy body disease, Parkinson's disease, frontotemporal degeneration, and vascular dementia, but Alzheimer's disease is the most common cause, accounting for 60–80% of cases. In 2013, I retired because I had developed MCI that was soon shown by biomarker testing to be due to early-stage Alzheimer's disease. I suddenly wore two hats – that of a retired physician with a lot of experience treating Alzheimer's disease and now of a person living with the same disorder [1].

There has been a lot of confusion and disagreement about the difference, if any, between Alzheimer's dementia and Alzheimer's disease. Until fairly recently, the terms were often used interchangeably. They both referred to dementia that was confirmed by autopsy to be associated with beta-amyloid plaques and tau-containing neurofibrillary tangles in the brain, the pathological hallmarks first described by Dr. Alois Alzheimer in 1906. When I was beginning to practice neurology in the 1980s, we referred to suspected Alzheimer's as senile dementia of the Alzheimer's type (SDAT). At that time there was no practical way to make a firm diagnosis during life, so we based our diagnosis on our experience with similar patients. Now there are good amyloid and tau biomarkers that have greatly increased the accuracy of diagnosis during life. These include brain PET scans, spinal fluid tests, and most recently, several very sensitive and specific blood tests that should soon be readily available.

Let's get back to the question: What is the difference between Alzheimer's dementia and Alzheimer's disease, and why is the distinction important? Alzheimer's disease is a continuum. At one extreme is dementia: cognitive impairment that interferes with doing everyday activities, getting more severe over time, and eventually causing death. The dementia phase of Alzheimer's lasts an average of 8–10 years. The first symptoms of cognitive problems usually don't interfere with daily activities. Work may still be possible. This phase is called MCI. Like dementia, MCI can be caused by other disorders, but in the presence of amyloid or tau biomarkers, Alzheimer's is almost always the cause. Dementia and MCI used to be all we cared about. But it is important to understand that the Alzheimer's pathology in the brain, the amyloid plaques and neurofibrillary tangles, begin appearing up to 20 years before the first symptoms of cognitive impairment. There is disagreement about when we should start calling this spectrum Alzheimer's disease. Those who would restrict the term to people with dementia or MCI argue that many people who have positive amyloid or tau biomarkers in middle age will never develop dementia. They might die of something else first, or they might have a resilient brain that resists these pathological changes. Why should we alarm these people who may never get Alzheimer's dementia? I understand this point of view. However, I think we should be receptive to the idea that the early, presymptomatic stage of Alzheimer's disease is likely to be the most effective time to attack the disease, to slow or even stop progression before any symptoms have occurred. We can already slow progression with evidence-based lifestyle modifications in midlife: getting adequate aerobic exercise, eating a Mediterranean-style diet, staying intellectually and socially engaged, getting adequate sleep, and managing cardiovascular risk factors such as high blood pressure, high cholesterol, diabetes, and smoking. New medications to treat Alzheimer's disease, such as the controversial FDA-approved aducanumab and similar anti-amyloid monoclonal antibodies, may turn out to be more effective if used early, during MCI, or even before cognitive symptoms are present. This is not a new idea. Although the anti-amyloid monoclonal antibody solanezumab failed to slow cognitive impairment in subjects with mild dementia due to Alzheimer's disease [2], a long-term, placebo-controlled study of solanezumab in older, cognitively normal subjects with positive amyloid PET scans has been underway since 2014 and will finish within the next year or two [3]. Two newer anti-amyloid monoclonal antibodies that are more effective in removing beta-amyloid, donanemab [4] and gantenerumab [5], are undergoing trials in subjects who do not yet have any cognitive impairment but have positive Alzheimer's biomarkers. They don't have Alzheimer's dementia yet. They don't even have MCI. But they are on the Alzheimer's continuum and are at high risk for developing dementia in the future. Recently, the anti-amyloid monoclonal antibody lecanemab was reported to reduce cognitive decline in subjects with either MCI or mild Alzheimer's dementia by 27% after 18 months [6]. Whether this is a clinically meaningful benefit can be debated, but it is the strongest evidence to date supporting a possible role for anti-amyloid drugs in the treatment of Alzheimer's, and there is already a trial underway of lecanemab using volunteers in the presymptomatic phase of the disease [7].

So, what's the difference? Alzheimer's dementia is the tip of the Alzheimer's disease iceberg. According to the *2023 Alzheimer's Disease Facts and Figures* [8], there are an estimated 6.7 million people over age 65 with Alzheimer's dementia now in the USA. That seems like a lot. But now let's add in the number with MCI and positive biomarkers for Alzheimer's, such as a positive amyloid PET scan. That group is estimated to contain more than five million people. These are people who are very likely to have Alzheimer's dementia within a few years. The prevalence of symptomatic Alzheimer's disease (dementia and MCI) is therefore about 12 million in the USA. Now let's add in the number of people with positive Alzheimer's biomarkers but no symptoms of cognitive impairment. That group was estimated to be 46 million in 2017 [9]. Now we have an estimate of nearly 58 million Americans who have Alzheimer's pathology in their brains. And most of them are young enough that intervention might successfully prevent dementia.

When should these presymptomatic people be identified and offered treatment? Certainly, the lifestyle modifications mentioned earlier should begin as early as possible, especially in those with a family history of Alzheimer's disease. For pharmaceutical interventions, we must follow the science as it unfolds. I would predict that our first successes will occur in research subjects who have a family history of Alzheimer's and who are within a few years of expected onset of cognitive impairment as identified by the presence of tau biomarkers. Waiting to treat Alzheimer's until dementia has set in is not likely to be successful. The horses are already out of the barn.

References

1   Gibbs DM. Early awareness of Alzheimer disease: A neurologist's personal perspective. *JAMA Neurology* 2019; 76: 249. https://doi.org/10.1001/jamaneurol.2018.4910. PMID: 30776065.

2   Honig LS, Vellas B, Woodward M, *et al.* Trial of solanezumab for mild dementia due to Alzheimer's disease. *N Engl J Med* 2018; 378: 321–330. https://doi.org/10.1056/NEJMoa1705971. PMID: 29365294.

3   Clinical trial of solanezumab for older individuals who may be at risk for memory loss (A4). https://clinicaltrials.gov/ct2/show/NCT02008357 (accessed May 12, 2022).

4   A donanemab (LY3002813) prevention study in participants with Alzheimer's disease (TRAILBLAZER-ALZ 3). https://clinicaltrials.gov/ct2/show/NCT05026866 (accessed May 12, 2022).

5   A study to evaluate the efficacy and safety of gantenerumab in participants at risk for or at the earliest stages of Alzheimer's disease (AD) (SKYLINE). https://clinicaltrials.gov/ct2/show/NCT05256134 (accessed May 12, 2022).

6   van Dyck CH, Swanson CJ, Aisen P, *et al.* Lecanemab in early Alzheimer's disease. *N Engl J Med* 2023; 388: 9–21. https://doi.org/10.1056/NEJMoa2212948.

7   AHEAD 3-45 Study: A study to evaluate efficacy and safety of treatment with lecanemab in participants with preclinical Alzheimer's disease and elevated amyloid and also in participants with early preclinical Alzheimer's disease and intermediate amyloid. https://clinicaltrials.gov/ct2/show/NCT04468659 (accessed December 29, 2022).

8   *2023 Alzheimer's Disease Facts and Figures.* www.alz.org/
     media/documents/alzheimers-facts-and-figures.pdf,
     pages 20–22 (accessed March 27, 2023, open access).
9   Brookmeyer R, Abdalla N, Kawas CH, Corrada MM.
     Forecasting the prevalence of preclinical and clinical
     Alzheimer's disease in the United States. *Alzheimers
     Dement* 2019; 14: 121–129. www.ncbi.nlm.nih.gov/pmc/
     articles/PMC5803316/ (accessed December 17, 2022,
     open access).

Note: This essay is based on my paper with the same title published in *Ageing
Research Reviews* with appropriate updates. https://doi.org/10.1016/j.arr.2022
.101779. Open access status has been granted by the publisher.

4 THE FIRST PATIENT WITH ALZHEIMER'S DISEASE

Recently, I came across an interesting paper from 2013 in *Lancet Neurology* that adds important genetic information about the case of Auguste D, the first patient diagnosed with what was later called Alzheimer's disease. She first came under the care of Dr. Alois Alzheimer at age 51 because of rapidly progressive memory loss, hallucinations, seizures, focal neurological signs including trouble speaking, and delusions that her husband was having an affair with the next-door neighbor, fears that were apparently unfounded. She died five years later, and Dr. Alzheimer was able to examine her brain under a microscope. He was surprised to find dark blobs outside of nerve cells and smaller dark tangles within the axons of nerve cells. He reported his findings in 1906 at the 37th Conference of South-West German Psychiatrists in Tübingen, but there was little interest from the audience. Soon other pathologists started seeing these dark extracellular blobs and intraneuronal twists in the brains of demented patients, later identified as beta-amyloid plaques and tau-containing neurofibrillary tangles. Dementia associated with these characteristic pathological findings came to be called Alzheimer's disease in his honor.

Until the 1970s, Alzheimer's disease referred only to demented patients such as Auguste D, less than 65 years of age who were later found to have amyloid plaques and neurofibrillary tangles. Alzheimer's disease was considered to be a type of presenile dementia. Demented patients older than 65 were felt to simply have senile dementia thought by many to be a normal consequence of aging. Over the last 40 years, the concept of Alzheimer's disease has evolved. While brain pathology is the same whether the cognitive problems start in the 40s or 70s, the genetics can be different. Three rare gene mutations cause an autosomal dominant form of early Alzheimer's. If you have just one copy of the *presenilin-1*, *presenilin-2*, or amyloid precursor protein (*APP*) gene mutation, you will almost certainly get Alzheimer's disease with rapidly progressive cognitive impairment starting in the 40s or 50s. Together, these three mutations account for less than 2% of all Alzheimer's cases and only 10% of those with symptoms before age 65. Other Alzheimer's risk genes, especially having two copies of *APOE-4*, can sometimes lead to early-onset disease as well. About 60% of people with late-onset Alzheimer's, beginning after age 65, have at least one copy of the *APOE-4* allele. This is an important point: *APOE-4* is the most important genetic risk factor for both early and late-onset Alzheimer's disease. Many other Alzheimer's risk genes have been found. With the exception of the determinative *presenilin* and *APP* gene mutations, having these risk genes simply increases the chance of getting Alzheimer's. Many people with these risk genes never develop dementia.

In a 2013 *Lancet Neurology* paper, Ulrich Müller and his colleagues at Justus Liebig University in Giessen, Germany reported their genetic analysis of histopathological tissue recovered from a single microscope slide prepared during Auguste D's original autopsy over a hundred years before [1]. They found that she had the *presenilin-1* mutation. Interestingly, she had two copies of the *APOE-3* allele, providing standard *APOE*-related risk. However, because of her *presenilin-1* mutation, she was doomed from birth to develop Alzheimer's disease at a relatively young age. Auguste had one child, a daughter named Thekla. She would have had a 50% chance of inheriting the *presenilin-1* mutation and developing early-onset Alzheimer's. Thekla died in 1940 at age 67, so it seems likely that she did not get the mutation.

References

1   Müller U, Winter P, Graeber MB. A presenilin 1 muta-
    tion in the first case of Alzheimer's disease. *Lancet Neurol*
    2013; 12: 129–130. https://doi.org/10.1016/S1474-4422(
    12)70307-1 (open access).

5 KIDNAPPED IN KINSHASA

Soon after I retired in 2013, I took a three-month course designed to prepare doctors and other health care workers for volunteer work in underserved parts of the developing world. In addition to the lectures on tropical diseases and practical training in free clinics and emergency rooms, we spent one full day undergoing training in personal security including how best to survive a kidnapping. We had lectures in the morning, and in the afternoon, we piled into off-road vehicles and entered a very realistic 10-acre training facility normally used by local police and fire departments. Our instructors were employees of a prominent non-governmental organization (NGO) that serves many of the most unstable regions of Africa and the Middle East. The driver of my vehicle in real life worked in a health clinic in the eastern part of the Democratic Republic of the Congo (DRC), one of the most dangerous areas for aid workers to operate. To add some authenticity, our driver pretended to speak no English, so our communication with her was only in French. I was the only one in our group with some high school French, so I served as translator. The lessons started out easy with how to deal with a policeman demanding a bribe. The scenarios escalated in intensity until finally our vehicle was stopped by armed men who put hoods over our heads and forced us into a small cabin while automatic weapon fire, presumably with blanks, was going on outside the walls. Of course, it wasn't real, but it was still a frightening experience. After debriefing about the shortcomings of our responses (we lost track of one of our compatriots who disappeared), I think we learned some useful lessons on how to respond in the very unlikely scenario of being unwillingly detained.

That moment came much sooner than I expected. Since 2008, I had been making yearly trips to Tanzania to teach neurology to medical students and resident doctors at the Kilimanjaro Christian Medical College in Moshi. English is the language of instruction from high school on in Tanzania, so I wasn't handicapped by my very limited knowledge of Swahili. My experiences in Tanzania were wonderful. I was welcomed by Tanzanian faculty and students as well as the local and ex-pat communities. I was never afraid, except once during an encounter with a green mamba, one of the deadliest snakes in the world. In 2014, after I had retired, I traveled to Mekelle University in Ethiopia with a delegation of faculty from my medical school, working out details for a possible collaboration. Again, my interactions with Ethiopians were very positive. I enjoyed giving a series of lectures and consulting on neurological patients on the wards and in clinic.

In 2015, I was invited to be on the faculty for a two-week course in neurology in Kinshasa, the capital of the DRC. The students taking the course were recently graduated neurologists and neuroscientists from all over sub-Saharan Africa. The course was arranged by the International Brain Research Organization, and the language of instruction was English. French is the language of higher education in the DRC, so some of our students had trouble with the lectures and discussion in English. Inevitably a bit of French was slipped in as well. I also gave a series of talks to the neurology and psychiatry residents at the University of Kinshasa Medical School and still another lecture at a separate neurology symposium in Kinshasa.

I was busy almost every day. I had looked forward to doing some sightseeing, but we had been warned not to leave the hotel without being accompanied by a Congolese

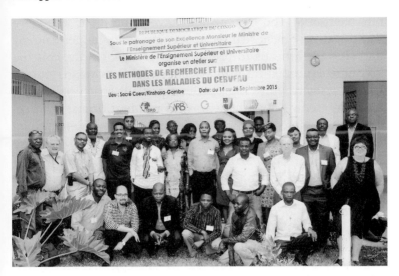

The faculty and students of the International Brain Research Organization neurology course in Kinshasa, DRC. I am third from the right in the first row standing. My friend from Gabon is in the suit immediately to my left.

local. On Sunday, one of the faculty from Gabon asked if I wanted to go on a walk with him. He is an imposing but extremely friendly man who actually has some research connections with the University of Oregon near where I live. Our hotel was located in the center of the city, surrounded almost entirely by government buildings. The streets were almost empty. We walked a mile or two taking in the sights and stopping at a market to buy some water and other supplies. We were less than a block from our hotel when an unmarked car with three men in plain clothes pulled up next to us. The man in the front passenger seat flashed a police badge, gruffly asked who we were, and demanded to see our passports. Fortunately, French is the native tongue of my Gabonese friend. He explained that both of us had left our passports in the hotel, and he offered to lead the "police" back to our hotel so we could produce our passports. The boss would have none of it. We were forced into the back seat by a burly guy who had left the car and stood behind us to prevent our escape. Oddly, this big guy who squeezed into the back seat with us was trying to calm us down while his boss in the front seat was yelling and threatening us. There was something almost comical about the whole episode, especially when they determined that I was an American and patted me down because "Americans always carry guns!" After about 30 minutes of driving around Kinshasa, while the boss in the front seat "inspected" our wallets and removed our euros and dollars but not our Congolese francs, we stopped on a relatively posh street where most of the houses had armed guards in front. The driver of our car got out and opened the trunk. This was the only time in the entire episode that I was frightened. I imagined that we might be killed and dumped in the trunk. But no, he was just covering his license plate with a cloth so we couldn't identify the car later. They then let us go with an admonition to keep our mouths shut. The car drove off with our money, and we immediately went to one of the nearby security guards to report the incident. He appeared sympathetic and directed us to the nearest police station to file a report, but my Gabonese friend decided it might be worse for us to report the theft if the thieves were indeed police officers. We eventually found our way back to our hotel on foot, keeping a wary eye pealed for other assailants. By this time, I was pretty sure that our kidnappers were not really police officers, but when we reported the episode to our hosts, we were told that they were almost certainly police. Political instability due to an upcoming presidential election had metastasized into the police department, threatening a longstanding system of patronage and graft. Also, we were told, other assailants would likely not have been as gentle with us and might indeed have killed us.

Later, looking back on this dramatic event, I wondered why I had not been more afraid and upset. My friend was visibly afraid while we sat in the back seat of the car being yelled at. Of course, it may just have been because he had prior experience with being robbed and assaulted. But I don't think that was the entire explanation. I was an extremely anxious and nervous child. I was still pretty anxious in my 20s. Anxiety ran in my family through my mother's side. I do think my security training helped, but I also wonder if my flattened affect was a result of my then early-stage Alzheimer's disease. I was still cognitively normal, and was still able to lecture from PowerPoint slides, even using a little French, but I was starting to have some flattening of my emotions. Apathy is a well-recognized, early symptom of Alzheimer's disease probably caused by Alzheimer's pathology in the prefrontal cortex [1]. A simplistic explanation would be to say that my ability to mount a flight or fight response to threat has been muted. Perhaps like my early loss of smell, this is not necessarily a bad thing.

References

1 van Dyck CH, Arnsten AFT, Padala PR, *et al.* Neurobiologic rationale for treatment of apathy in Alzheimer's disease with methylphenidate. *Am J Geriatr Psychiatry* 2021; 29: 51–62 https://doi.org/10.1016/j.jagp.2020.04.026 (open access).

6 SMELL, DISGUST, AND ALZHEIMER'S

The earliest neuropathological changes of Alzheimer's disease, the beta-amyloid plaques, usually appear first in the olfactory parts of the brain including the olfactory bulb, anterior olfactory nucleus, and entorhinal cortex [1]. I totally lost my ability to smell several years before I developed any measurable cognitive impairment. Almost all people with Alzheimer's have at least some impairment of olfaction, but most are not aware of it unless tested, probably because it comes on so gradually.

I am often asked what it's like to not be able to smell. Of course, there are downsides. Food all tastes pretty much the same, not bad, but not very interesting. I really miss the smell of bacon frying in the pan. I wouldn't be able to smell a gas leak, so there are safety issues. But there are a few advantages. I have no trouble eating the bitter vegetables such as kale and Brussels sprouts that are very high in flavonols and are important components of the MIND diet [2]. I don't waste money on expensive wines. I can't smell the spray of a skunk. And I'm not grossed out by messy dog poop cleanup or changing a grandchild's diaper. By the time my sense of smell was completely gone, I started to be aware of something else. I don't get disgusted anymore. At first, I thought this was just because I could no longer smell disgusting things, but it seems to be more complicated than that. I find that I have become a more tolerant person. I will engage a homeless person in conversation, something I'm ashamed to admit I would not have done in the past. I don't necessarily think I am more empathetic.

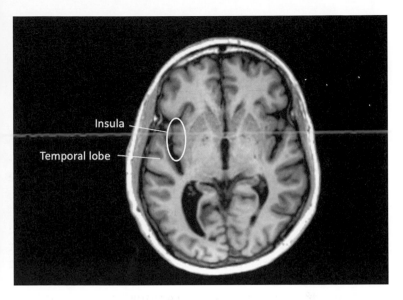

A recent MRI of my brain showing the location of the insula and temporal lobe.

People with Alzheimer's usually have trouble with empathy. I think it is just that the protective barrier of disgust is no longer working, and maybe that results in something resembling empathy.

The insula is the main part of our brain that processes disgust. It is located deep in the brain at the bottom of the lateral sulcus. It lights up on a functional MRI scan when a research subject sniffs a foul odor. It even lights up when a subject watches the facial expression of someone else smelling a foul odor [3]. Although amyloid plaques and neurofibrillary tangles eventually appear in the insula, it is usually not directly affected until later in the disease.

Don't worry, there will not be a quiz. I show this schematic just to illustrate how complex the pathways are connecting the olfactory epithelium in the nose (upper left) to the insular cortex (on right, second box from top).

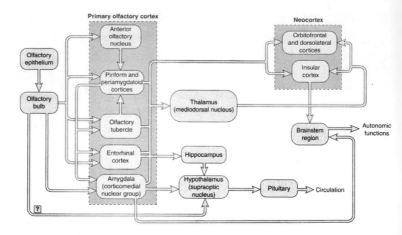

From Christopher H. Hawkes and Richard L. Doty, *Smell and Taste Disorders* 2018, Cambridge University Press, p. 20 [4].

As shown in the MRI image of my brain on page 27, my insula still looks pretty good. There is little if any atrophy unlike in the adjacent temporal lobe. My inability to register disgust probably lies elsewhere in this labyrinth of neuronal pathways, but that's OK with me. I am actually quite happy to have a life without disgust.

References

1   Serrano-Pozo A, Frosch MP, Masliah E, Hyman BT. Neuropathological alterations in Alzheimer disease. *Cold Spring Harb Perspect Med* 2011; 1(1): a006189. https://doi.org/10.1101/cshperspect.a006189.   PMID: 22229116; PMCID: PMC3234452 (open access version).

2   Holland TM, Agarwal P, Wang Y, *et al.* Dietary flavonols and risk of Alzheimer's dementia. *Neurology* 2020; 94: e1749–e1756 (open access version available at www.ncbi.nlm.nih.gov/pmc/articles/PMC7282875).

3   Wicker B, Keysers C, Plailly J, *et al.* Both of us disgusted in my insula: The common neural basis seeing and

feeling disgust. *Neuron* 2003; 40: 655–664. https://doi
.org/10.1016/s0896-6273(03)00679-2. PMID: 14642287
(open access version).

4   Hawkes CH, Doty RL. *Smell and Taste Disorders*.
Cambridge: Cambridge University Press, 2018, p. 20.

7 APOLIPOPROTEIN-4 (APOE-4)
Bad for the Brain and Bad for the Heart

At some point while I was a medical student in the 1970s, I had my cholesterol checked. I think it was part of a pedagogical exercise, and as I recall, only the total cholesterol was measured. Surprisingly, the cholesterol level was near the upper limit of normal. Too many burgers and fries, said Lois. I laughed it off. There wasn't much heart disease in the family. One of my grandfathers died of a heart attack, a myocardial infarction, but he was in his mid-70s. I was in my 20s and invincible. As I grew older, my cholesterol levels, especially the low-density lipoprotein (LDL) cholesterol, crept higher, and the upper limits of normal were revised down so that by the time I was in my 40s, my cholesterol was unambiguously elevated. By the time I was in my 50s, I was taking medications to keep my cholesterol levels and blood pressure under control. As the years went by, the doses of these medications continued to climb. My hyperlipidemia and hypertension have always been a bit of a puzzle to me, but they have both been manageable with medications and diet.

As I have previously mentioned, I inadvertently learned that I have two copies of the *APOE*-4 allele in 2012 while pursuing DNA testing for genealogical purposes. Apolipoprotein E is an important carrier protein for cholesterol in the blood. The gene coding for apolipoprotein E comes in three isoforms, *APOE-2*, *APOE-3*, and *APOE-4* (By convention, the gene is written in italics, and the protein produced by transcription of that gene into mRNA with subsequent translation into protein is written in normal script). Having one copy of the *APOE-4* allele increases the risk of getting Alzheimer's disease by about three-fold, and having two copies increases the risk by about 12-fold, although one study in which the diagnosis of Alzheimer's was confirmed at autopsy suggests that the risk of Alzheimer's due to *APOE-4* is actually much higher [1]. *APOE-3*, the most common allele, confers neutral risk, and *APOE-2*, a relatively rare allele, confers substantial protection against Alzheimer's, especially when two copies are present.

But why should a gene coding for a cholesterol-carrying lipoprotein have anything to do with the risk of getting Alzheimer's? When Dr. Allen Roses and his team at Duke University discovered this connection in the 1990s, his work was initially dismissed. It did not seem to fit the paradigm of the time, the amyloid hypothesis. He had trouble getting research funding, so he was forced to take out a loan secured against his home to support his research [2]. Eventually he was vindicated, and *APOE-4* is now recognized as the most important genetic risk factor for Alzheimer's disease (aside from rare mutations in one of three genes, amyloid precursor protein (*APP*), *presenilin-1* (*PSEN1*), or *presenilin-2* (*PSEN2*), that cause early-onset, auto-somal-dominant Alzheimer's).

It turns out that cholesterol bound to apolipoprotein cir-culating in the blood cannot get into the brain because it cannot cross the blood brain barrier. However, cholesterol and apolipoproteins are also synthesized in the brain, pri-marily in astrocytes, and then transferred to other cell types in the brain. They don't have to cross the blood brain barrier. This brain cholesterol is closely regulated. It is needed for normal brain function, but too much can interfere with functions of several types of brain cells including microglia, the inflammatory cells of the brain, and oligodendrocytes, cells that make the myeline sheaths around neuronal axons. APOE-4 causes dysregulation of cholesterol metabolism in the brain, and this is thought to be at the core of increased risk of developing Alzheimer's disease [3].

Not surprisingly, carrying the APOE-4 allele, especially two copies, also increases the risk for cardiovascular disease. In a recent meta-analysis of 33 studies looking at the role of the various apolipoprotein isoforms on risk for myocardial infarction (MI), MI was more likely in those with at least one copy of APOE-4 (compared to APOE-3-associated risk) and less likely in those carrying the APOE-2 allele. Research subjects carrying APOE-4 have higher baseline LDL cholesterol and triglycerides, and they have a reduced response to the cholesterol-lowering effects of statins [4].

Bottom line? The APOE-4 allele is a risk factor for both heart and brain disease. Carrying the APOE-4 allele, especially two copies, increases the risk of Alzheimer's and cardiovascular disease, but it doesn't mean that you are doomed to get them. It is possible to reduce the risk by adopting healthy heart and brain lifestyle modifications. Get daily aerobic exercise. Eat a Mediterranean-style diet such as the MIND diet. Stop smoking. Get at least seven hours of sleep per night. Control hypertension, diabetes, sleep apnea, obesity, and hyperlipidemia if present. And specifically for Alzheimer's prevention, stay socially and intellectually engaged.

References

1   Reiman   EM,   Arboleda-Velasquez   JF,   Quiroz YT, et al. Exceptionally low likelihood of Alzheimer's dementia in APOE2 homozygotes from a 5,000-person neuropathological study. *Nat Commun* 2020; 11: 667. https://doi.org/10.1038/s41467-019-14279-8 (open access).

2   Roberts S. Allen Roses, who upset common wisdom on cause of Alzheimer's, dies at 73. *New York Times* October 5, 2016. www.nytimes.com/2016/10/06/science/allen-roses-who-upset-common-wisdom-on-cause-of-alzhei mers-dies-at-73.html (open access).

3   Jeong W, Lee H, Cho S, Seo J. ApoE4-induced cholesterol dysregulation and its brain cell type-specific implications in the pathogenesis of Alzheimer's disease. *Mol Cells* 2019; 42: 739–746. https://doi.org/10.14348/molcells.2019.0200 (open access).

4   Shao A, Shi J, Liang Z, *et al.* Meta-analysis of the association between apolipoprotein E polymorphism and risks of myocardial infarction. *BMC Cardiovasc Disord* 2022; 22: 126. https://doi.org/10.1186/s12872-022-02566-0 (open access).

8 LOST IN THE FOG OF ALZHEIMER'S

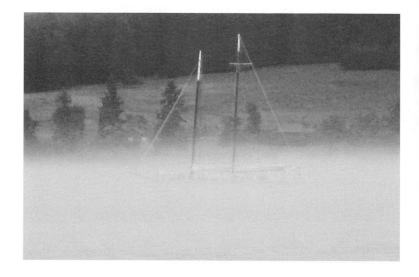

Getting literally lost in the fog is a terrifying experience. It happened to me about 30 years ago while sailing in the San Juan Islands, an archipelago that lies between Vancouver Island in British Columbia and northwest Washington State. We left shore with clear skies, but about an hour later a fog bank suddenly rolled in limiting visibility to no more than 50 feet. Our chartered boat had neither GPS nor radar, so we were almost instantly disoriented. Our only source of reference was the compass. I found it surprisingly difficult to steer a straight course by compass alone as every time I took my eyes off the dial, the boat would head off in another direction. We inched along, blowing our foghorn frequently and listening for the horns of other boats nearby. One of those horns was on a very large ferry that seemed to be getting closer all the time despite our frantic attempts to head away from it. The fog finally lifted after an hour, but I think those 60 minutes were among the most stressful of my life.

The fog of Alzheimer's is a commonly used metaphor, and I think it's a pretty good one. It refers to the loss of mental acuity, disorientation, and forgetfulness that are common in Alzheimer's. But one aspect of the metaphor that is not emphasized is that like the fog bank on the ocean, the fog of Alzheimer's can come and go. It does for me. Sometimes there is an obvious cause such as running a fever, getting too tired, or having a second glass of wine. On the day after I got my second Covid-19 vaccination, I was not mentally sharp and had trouble concentrating despite not having any other side effects. Once or twice a week on first awakening in the morning, I think I am in my child-hood bedroom. It only takes a few seconds to get reoriented, and it actually is a pleasant rather than scary experience. Sometimes the fog comes in for no apparent reason, lasts a few minutes or a few hours, and then goes away. I wonder what is behind these mysterious, seemingly unprovoked but temporary episodes of cognitive impairment.

In December 2018, after receiving four doses of the anti-amyloid monoclonal antibody aducanumab in a phase 3 trial, I suffered severe swelling and bleeding in my brain requiring ICU care and several months to return to my cognitive baseline [1]. These episodes are called amyloid-related imaging abnormalities or ARIA. During the recovery period, I had a marked increase in the frequency and sever-ity of my foggy spells. Abnormal brain wave activity is very common in people with Alzheimer's disease, and seizures are not particularly rare. I wondered if the damage done by the swelling and bleeding in my brain was provoking seizures. Seizures are relatively common in people with

Alzheimer's, and electroencephalograms (EEG) are almost always abnormal. At the least, the EEG shows abnormal slowing of brain wave activity in Alzheimer's. Some people have frank seizures and corresponding epileptiform sharp waves on their EEGs. These sharp waves can also be seen in others without obvious epileptic events. I asked my neurologist to check an EEG, and sure enough, it showed frequent epileptiform sharp waves, worse in the left frontal-temporal region of my brain but appearing occasionally on the right as well. In addition, the background rhythm was slow bilaterally but more so on the left. I took the anticonvulsant medication levetiracetam (Keppra) for a few months, and the foggy spells markedly improved. We repeated the EEG in a year. The background electrical activity was slower than normal because of my Alzheimer's disease, but the sharp waves had almost completely resolved along with the frequent foggy spells. In my case, the foggy spells were probably due, at least in part, to non-convulsive seizures. They were decreased by an anticonvulsant that was needed for only a few months as my brain healed from the episode of ARIA.

The foggy spells of Alzheimer's, the episodic confusion and disorientation, can have many causes. The common occurrence of sundowning, an increase in confusion throughout the evening hours in people with Alzheimer's, is thought to be due to the decrease in sensory stimulation at night. Concomitant illnesses especially if associated with fever, hypoxia (low blood oxygen), or hypoglycemia (low blood sugar) may present as an altered mental state, a foggy spell, often before other symptoms are present. Complex partial seizures (seizures originating in the temporal or frontal lobes without limb jerking or other motor manifestations) typically last up to three minutes, but a state of confusion may persist for an hour or more. Seizures of all types are relatively common in people with Alzheimer's, occurring up to seven times more often than in similarly aged people without dementia [2]. Any change in the frequency or quality of foggy spells in an Alzheimer's patient should prompt the treating physician to search for a remedial cause.

References

1   VandeVrede L, Gibbs DM, Koestler M, *et al.* Symptomatic amyloid-related imaging abnormalities in an APOE ε4/ε4 patient treated with aducanumab. *Alzheimers Dement* 2020; 12: e12101. https://doi.org/10.1002/dad2.12101 (open access).

2   Irizarry MC, Jin S, He F, *et al.* Incidence of new-onset seizures in mild to moderate Alzheimer disease. *Arch Neurol* 2012; 69: 368–372. https//doi.org/10.1001/archneurol.2011.830 (public access version available at www.ncbi.nlm.nih.gov/PMC3622046).

9 MY FATHER'S "STUFF"

My father, Zack Gibbs, was 44 when I was born in 1951. He died of cancer 16 years later at age 60. Throughout his life he was a tinkerer. He liked to build things from scratch, something he got from his father who grew up on a farm. Both of them made toys for me. Unlike his father who made me things from wood, my dad loved designing and building electrical gadgets. I think he got his start in electronics from working in the 1930s as a technician for Professor Donald Menzel, the first director of the Harvard Observatory and a distant cousin. Among other things, my father helped Professor Menzel build a solar mask that allowed the study of the sun's corona. Later, he designed seismographic instruments for oil prospecting in Arkansas and forecasting rock bursts in a gold mine in Lakeshore, Ontario. In the early 1950s, he designed, built, and maintained radiation equipment for a cancer clinic in Los Angeles.

When I was young, he had a small company that manufactured an electrostatic flocking machine, a totally new concept at the time. Until then, flocking of garments and greeting cards was done by applying glue through a stencil or silkscreen, and then dusting the flock onto the glue. Not surprisingly, the flock lay down flat. In my father's machine, the flock first passed through a high voltage, direct current field that created a polarizing charge on each particle of flock so that when it landed in the glue, it stood on end. This was the beginning of fuzzy-feeling flock.

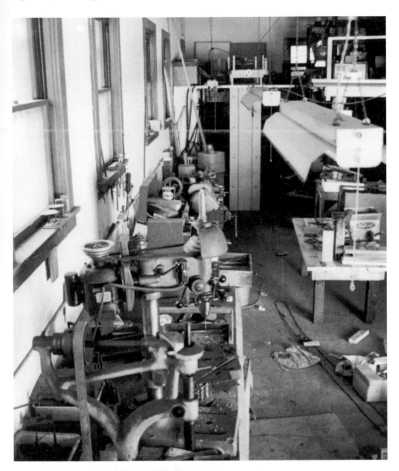

My father's workshop on Avenue 50 in Highland Park.

I loved tagging along when he worked in his workshop near Occidental College in Highland Park, California. I'm not sure what the original purpose of the old building was, but it had a large room with a concrete floor that served as the workshop and many rooms that probably had once been offices, but which he used to store his extra "stuff." He collected anything electronic. There were hundreds of

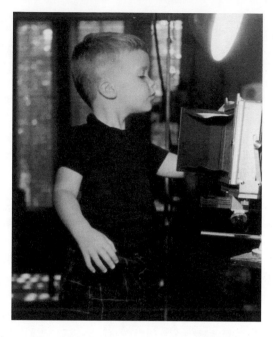

Me checking out an old portrait camera under my father's supervision.

meters, vacuum tubes, power supplies, old TV sets, wire recorders (a precursor of the tape recorder), radios, and speakers. It was a child's dream come true to hunt through these rooms of stuff looking for treasures while my father was working. We would build things together using things literally off the shelf. We never had to order anything.

There were also many cameras of all shapes, sizes, and vintage. He got me started taking photographs at a very early age, a hobby I have treasured throughout my life. There is no doubt that my life in science and medicine got its start from my father, his workshop, and his glorious collection of stuff.

There may have been a darker aspect to my father's workshop. In addition to the many rooms full of stuff, there were at least five garages in the back that he had also filled with unwanted, derelict equipment including a broken-down washing machine. At the time, my father was considered to be a bit eccentric, but today he would almost certainly be diagnosed as having hoarding disorder. Our garage at home was also full of clutter. There were at least two drill presses, a lathe, many meters, and more boxes of miscellaneous stuff. I suspect the acquisition of his workshop in Highland Park was in part due to my mother's desire to keep stuff from invading our home more than it already had.

And then there is the possible Alzheimer's connection. Hoarding disorder is seen fairly commonly in people with moderate to advanced Alzheimer's dementia, but it is generally felt to be the result of dementia. My father died early at age 60. Despite having at least one copy of the *APOE-4* allele (because I have two copies), he had no evidence of cognitive impairment during his life. Could hoarding be an early warning of Alzheimer's such as loss of smell? Recall that I began to lose my sense of smell nearly ten years before being diagnosed with MCI due to Alzheimer's pathology. There is surprisingly little in the medical literature addressing this question. Hoarding disorder is strongly associated with other psychiatric disorders such as major depressive disorder, major anxiety disorder, and obsessive-compulsive disorder, but only weakly associated with mild cognitive impairment [1]. As far as I could tell, there has been no attempt to look for biomarkers of presymptomatic Alzheimer's disease in subjects with hoarding disorder.

Hoarding disorder or not, my father's vast collection of "stuff" was indeed a dream come true for a young boy with a curious mind. I think my mother saw it all as junk, and in fact she called in a junk removal service to get rid of most of the stuff after he died, but otherwise the "stuff" was a pleasure for my father and a source of adventure for me.

References

1   Vieir LS, Guastello A, Nguyen B, *et al.* Identifying psychiatric and neurological comorbidities associated with hoarding disorder through network analysis. *J Psychiatr Res* 2022; 156: 16–24. https://doi.org/10.1016/j.jpsychires.2022.09.037 (open access).

10 FACE BLINDNESS DURING A PANDEMIC

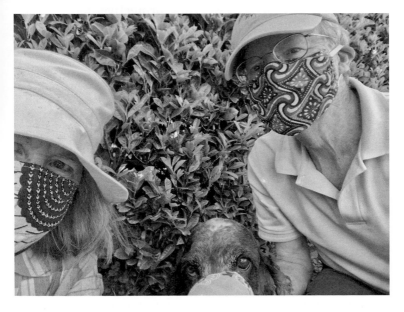

Selfie of Lois, Jack, and me masked up at the beginning of the Covid-19 pandemic.

One morning during the peak of the Covid-19 pandemic, I was walking my dog Jack in our neighborhood, and I encountered a blonde woman walking her dog while pushing a toddler in a stroller. I stopped to chat, asking her how old her son was now, and she responded amiably. About a year and a half before, three women on our block gave birth within a month of each other. One woman has blonde hair and two have dark hair. They all have dogs.

As soon as we had ended our chat and I was walking on, I realized that she had the wrong dog. The blonde on our block has a black lab, and this dog was some kind of curly-haired terrier. I then realized that the woman I had approached was a complete stranger, not one of my neighbors.

On the face of it, this wouldn't be a particularly noteworthy incident, given the context of the Covid-19 pandemic that had us all wearing protective face masks. It became a common, shared experience, these awkward social moments in which we've failed to recognize people we know, or we've been on the receiving end of someone we know looking right past us as if we're strangers. But the moment held more for me.

I am a retired neurologist with Alzheimer's disease. Being a neurologist with a neurological disorder has provided me with some special insights. For example, seeing beta-amyloid on my first amyloid PET scan located not only in the prefrontal cortex and precuneus but also in olfactory processing centers such as the piriform cortex and orbital frontal cortex was really exciting because it provided a logical explanation for the early loss of smell I have described previously. The PET scans also gave me some hints as to the cause of my trouble recognizing my neighbors.

Face blindness, or prosopagnosia, is a neurological condition resulting in trouble identifying human faces. It is usually caused by damage to the fusiform gyrus in the posterior temporal lobe and anterior portion of the occipital lobe. Oliver Sacks famously introduced this condition to popular culture in his 1987 book *The Man Who Mistook His Wife for a Hat*. Dr. Sacks wrote about his own, severe face blindness in a fascinating, August 23, 2010 article in *The New Yorker* [1]. One of my neurology colleagues has such severe face blindness that she needs to hear someone speak before reliably making an identification. Like Oliver Sacks, she's had it all her life. Up to 2.5% of people are born with congenital face blindness, mostly inherited in an autosomal dominant pattern. Acquired face blindness may be caused by head trauma, strokes, or tumors affecting the fusiform gyrus. A more insidious form of face blindness occurs in many people with Alzheimer's disease, even in the early stages. The tau-containing neurofibrillary tangles of Alzheimer's disease usually first occur in the medial portion of the anterior temporal lobes. With time, these neurofibrillary tangles can spread backward into the fusiform gyrus.

Although my cognitive impairment is still mild to moderate, I have been having increasing trouble recognizing

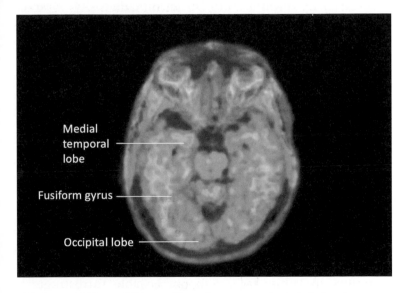

This is my 2018 tau-PET scan (done for a research study) showing abnormal tau protein (red and yellow colors) extending from the medial temporal lobes posteriorly into the region of the fusiform gyrus. Courtesy of Dr. Gil Rabinovici, UCSF Memory and Aging Center. (A black and white version of this figure will appear in some formats. For the color version, refer to the plate section.)

faces, even of people I know well. Many of my neighbors are hard for me to recognize until I hear their voices or see the dog they are walking. This was all the more problematic during the Covid-19 pandemic because of the universal mask wearing when out and about. On the other hand, I suspect that many normal people were having some trouble recognizing faces covered by masks. Before the pandemic, I would often be embarrassed by not recognizing or misidentifying an acquaintance while walking my dog. During the pandemic, not so much. It seems that most walkers like me were less inclined to greet passers-by, perhaps because none of us were quite sure who we were greeting. Our masks were covering important facial features used for facial recognition. A study from York University in Toronto and Ben-Gurion University in Israel confirmed this by demonstrating quantitative and qualitative changes in the visual processing of masked faces that could have significant effects on activities of daily living [2]. Perhaps we were all experiencing a degree of face blindness.

The ability to accurately identify other people by recognizing their faces is important to our social, emotional, and cultural behaviors. Our brains appear to learn how to recognize the faces of other people of our race during childhood. A study in 2019 showed that there is a critical period for this learning. Children learn how to recognize faces of the group they are raised with, up until about age 12 [3]. White children will become adept at distinguishing White faces, but unless they are exposed to other racial faces, they will have trouble distinguishing people of other races. Similarly, an Asian child raised in an Asian country without exposure to White faces will not be able to distinguish White faces. An Asian child adopted and raised in a predominantly White country will distinguish White faces but not Asian faces. A child who grows up in a racially heterogeneous setting will be able to distinguish faces of all of those races. This learning process slows down and is gone by age 12.

To me, this suggests that there may be pathways in the brain, probably in the fusiform gyrus, that are developing new neuronal connections during childhood as we learn what makes one face look different from another, but that this plasticity is lost by age 12. It strikes me that while facemasks are drawing our attention to the subject of face blindness, more relevant may be the impact of our children's social exposure that supports how they see others, literally, in our diverse communities.

In the meantime, if I hope to avoid awkward moments on my dog walks, then I'll need to attend closely to those masked faces to overcome my combined disadvantage of neurological face blindness and masked face blindness, the first caused by abnormalities of the brain and the second simply due to the blocking of visual cues. My best option may be to pay closer attention to the dogs. Even for me, pets are easy to identify because of shape, size, color of coat, and sometimes temperament or behavior. I'll keep my eye on those canine companions from now on, but I'll also need to expand my mental dog gallery now to include that curly terrier and his friendly human companion with the baby stroller. Next time we pass on the street, we'll be strangers no more.

References

1 Sacks O. Face-blind – why are some of us terrible at recognizing faces? *The New Yorker* 2010 (Aug 23). www .newyorker.com/magazine/2010/08/30/face-blind (open access).
2 Freud E, Stajduhar A, Rosenbaum RS, *et al.* The COVID-19 pandemic masks the way people perceive faces. *Sci Rep* 2020; 10: 22344. https://doi.org/10.1038/s41598-020-78986-9 (open access).

3   McKone E, Wan L, Pidcock M, *et al.* A critical period for faces: Other-race face recognition is improved by childhood but not adult social contact. *Sci Rep* 2019; 9: 12820. https://doi.org/10.1038/s41598-019-49202-0 (open access).

Note: This essay was previously published in a similar form online in *Scientific American* on April 21, 2021: www.scientificamerican.com/article/what-its-like-to-have-face-blindness-during-the-pandemic/?previewid=8D032288-E26E-45B5-9B0B5C09C6733ADA.

11 BIOMARKERS FOR ALZHEIMER'S DISEASE

Early in my career as a general neurologist, there was no way to accurately make a diagnosis of Alzheimer's disease in a living patient. The only way then to know for sure that a patient had Alzheimer's was to see the classic amyloid plaques and tau-containing neurofibrillary tangles in the brain at autopsy. We could exclude some potentially treatable mimics of Alzheimer's such as certain brain tumors, strokes, and so-called normal pressure hydrocephalus with CT or MRI scans, but we really had little help in distinguishing the several types of progressive dementia due either to Alzheimer's disease, vascular dementia, Lewy body dementia, Parkinson's disease, or frontotemporal dementia. In the late 1980s and early 1990s, it really didn't matter much if we couldn't tell them apart because we had no treatment for any of these disorders. Then in 1996, donepezil (Aricept) was approved for the treatment of Alzheimer's disease. Suddenly it became more important to be able to be as accurate as possible in our diagnosis of dementia. Donepezil provides some cognitive benefit in many patients with Alzheimer's as well in some with Lewy body dementia [1], but it sometimes makes patients with frontotemporal dementia worse. We neurologists had to hone our diagnostic skills. Alzheimer's disease often, but not always, presents first with impairment of verbal memory. Lewy body dementia is classically associated with early visual hallucinations. Frontotemporal dementia usually begins much earlier than Alzheimer's, and it often causes marked personality changes that precede cognitive decline. However, not every patient who came to autopsy turned out to have the cause of dementia that we had diagnosed during life. We needed better biomarkers, tests that directly or indirectly helped determine what type of dementia was present while the patient was still alive.

Brain imaging tests such as CT and MRI scans can be helpful biomarkers for frontotemporal dementia because of the typical atrophy of the frontal and temporal lobes sparing more posterior parts of the brain. For other types of dementia, these imaging tests are not as helpful, although they may be important to rule out tumors, strokes, and hydrocephalus (excess fluid in the brain). Over the last ten years or so, PET scans that can image beta-amyloid plaques and tau-containing tangles have been developed and are now clinically available. These scans can be very useful in confirming the diagnosis of Alzheimer's and staging the severity of the disease in research settings. However, they are very expensive and often not covered by insurance, presenting barriers for clinical use outside of research.

Measurements of beta-amyloid and tau in spinal fluid have been useful tools in confirming a diagnosis of Alzheimer's, but these tests require a spinal tap that may be uncomfortable. There has been an extensive search for blood tests for forms of beta-amyloid and tau that are specific for Alzheimer's disease and that correlate with the progression of dementia. It seems that a new test is described every few months that is more selective and sensitive than the others. Currently, the leader is an assay for p-tau217 (tau protein phosphorylated at position 217) [2]. P-tau217 can be detected in blood plasma well before the onset of cognitive impairment, and it continues to climb as Alzheimer's progresses while also correlating with plasma beta-amyloid levels. Importantly, it is not elevated in other tauopathies such as frontotemporal dementia, progressive supranuclear palsy, corticobasal degeneration, and chronic traumatic encephalopathy (the early dementia seen in some athletes and soldiers who have suffered multiple head injuries [3]). Thus, the blood test for p-tau217 seems to be very sensitive and specific for Alzheimer's disease.

Most of these blood tests are not yet commercially available, but they are already being used to screen subjects for clinical trials of potential therapeutic drugs [4]. This is becoming increasingly important as it seems likely that the effective treatment of Alzheimer's disease may require administering drugs before symptoms of cognitive impairment have begun. In the near future, the ideal biomarkers may help us define the best time to start treatment. If we wait for the onset of cognitive impairment, it will probably be too late.

References

1 Mori E, Ikeda M, Nagai R, *et al.* Long-term donepezil use for dementia with Lewy bodies: Results from an open-label extension of Phase III trial. *Alzheimers Res Ther* 2015; 7: 5. https://doi.org/10.1186/s13195-014-0081-2. PMID: 25713600; PMCID: PMC4338564 (open access).

2 Milà-Alomà M, Ashton NJ, Shekari M, *et al.* Plasma p-tau231 and p-tau217 as state markers of amyloid-β pathology in preclinical Alzheimer's disease. *Nat Med* 2022; 28: 1797–1801. https://doi.org/10.1038/s41591-022-01925-w (open access).

3 Priemer DS, Iacono D, Rhodes CH, *et al.* Chronic traumatic encephalopathy in the brains of military personnel. *N Engl J Med* 2022; 386: 2169–2177. https://doi.org/10.1056/NEJMoa2203199.

4 Hansson O, Edelmayer RM, Boxer AL, *et al.* The Alzheimer's Association appropriate use recommendations for blood biomarkers in Alzheimer's disease. *Alzheimers Dement* 2022; 18: 2669–2686. https://doi.org/10.1002/alz.12756. Epub 2022 Jul 31. PMID: 35908251 (open access).

12 OLFACTORY IMPAIRMENT IN COVID-19 AND ALZHEIMER'S

Recently, I read a fascinating article in the *New York Times* by restaurant critic Tejal Rao about her sudden loss of smell due to Covid-19 last year:

> I noted that moment as it happened to me, stepping into the shower at my home in Los Angeles. At first, I mistook the lack of aromas for a new smell, a curious smell I couldn't identify — was it the water itself? the stone tiles? — before realizing it was just a blank, a cushion of space between me and my world [1].

At the time of her writing, she had experienced partial recovery of her sense of smell, an improvement that she attributes at least in part to smell training.

After loss of smell because of aging, infections of the nose and sinuses by a variety of viruses and bacteria are the most common cause of decreased ability to smell. We have all experienced this as a symptom of the common cold. Most of the time the anosmia (loss of smell) or hyposmia (decreased smell) is temporary and is mostly due to obstruction of the nasal passages, a stuffy nose. The odors just can't reach the olfactory receptors located high up in the sinuses. Some viruses and even some bacteria have an affinity for the olfactory receptors in the sinuses and even the olfactory nerve that carries smell information to the brain. The impairment of smell due to these infections can be long lasting and sometimes permanent. Almost everyone who tests positive for the Covid-19 virus has olfactory impairment when tested. It is only occasionally associated with a stuffy nose, is usually sudden in onset, and frequently, is the very first symptom [2].

In contrast to Covid-19 induced anosmia, the loss of smell seen in Alzheimer's disease is insidious in onset and slowly progressive. It does not go away. As in my case, it can begin ten years or more before the onset of cognitive impairment. Many if not most people with Alzheimer's disease don't even notice the loss because it progresses so slowly. I don't think I would have paid any attention to it had it not been for the illusory odors I experienced, the scent of baking bread mixed with perfume. These phantosmias, as they are called, would just come out of the blue. My sense of smell gradually disappeared entirely over four or five years. The phantosmias continued but became less frequent, finally disappearing altogether a few years ago.

Why does the loss of smell often improve after recovery from Covid-19 whereas the olfactory problems in Alzheimer's only get worse with time? We are still learning more about Covid-19 almost every day, but the answer probably involves the location and type of injury. In Covid, the virus attacks olfactory receptors in the sinuses, the olfactory nerve, and probably the olfactory bulb, the first center in the brain for processing olfactory signals. The Covid-19 virus appears to cause inflammation and swelling in these areas, and this inflammation probably resolves as the infection runs its course. By contrast, smell loss in Alzheimer's disease is due to damage of not only the olfactory bulb but also other olfactory centers higher in the brain such as the piriform cortex and orbitofrontal cortex. Amyloid plaques and tau-containing neurofibrillary tangles can be found in these sites before there has been any loss of memory or other cognitive impairments due to Alzheimer's. The damage progresses in these centers over the years and is probably irreversible.

For me, the very gradual loss of my ability to smell due to Alzheimer's has been relatively easy to adapt to. I like a lot of spice in my food because otherwise there isn't much taste, and I don't have to buy expensive wine, they all taste the same to me now. I don't mind picking up dog poop or other smelly jobs. On the other hand, I sometimes really miss the aroma of bacon frying in the pan or an apple pie just out of the oven.

A few months ago, I came down with a Covid-19 infection despite being up-to-date on all my vaccinations and boosters, and wearing a mask in public. Fortunately, I was only sick for a few days, probably because I was well-immunized. I knew I likely wouldn't see any effect on my sense of smell because it has been totally absent due to Alzheimer's for years. However, I did notice a change in my sense of taste. Of course, my sense of taste has been diminished because I can't smell, but what is left of my ability to taste has been stable for several years. On the first day of fevers and chills from Covid-19, I noticed a shift in taste such that things that once tasted sweet either had no taste or tasted sour. Chocolate no longer had an appealing taste. Orange juice tasted sour and salty. Impairment of smell and/or taste is common in people during Covid infection, occurring in about half of subjects, but it usually returns with time. Indeed, within a week or ten days, my sense of taste returned to baseline.

Another thing affected by Covid was my cognitive ability. It wasn't just the fever. I had to ask Lois what my cell phone number was on a day when I was otherwise on the mend. I know my cell number now, several months after the Covid infection, but I still am not as sharp as I want to be. The Covid virus easily enters the brain, even in mild cases. Neurological symptoms commonly include headache and mild cognitive impairment (Covid fog), but more severe neurological complications including ataxia and strokes have been reported. Interestingly, Covid infection appears to slightly increase the chance of developing Alzheimer's dementia in the year following infection. The effect is small, and it is most pronounced in women over 85 years old. These women are about 1.9 times more likely to be diagnosed with Alzheimer's than those who did not have Covid [3].

I could find surprisingly little information about the possible effects of Covid infection in those who already have Alzheimer's disease. There are many papers looking at the cognitive effects of isolation during the early days of the pandemic, but there is almost nothing that addresses my most burning question: Are those of us who already have Alzheimer's likely to have an acceleration of cognitive decline if we get sick with Covid? I would guess that the answer would be yes, but I haven't found any high-quality studies that specifically address the issue. It may turn out to be difficult to distinguish acceleration of cognitive decline due to Covid from accelerated decline due to other causes, but I'll keep checking the Covid/Alzheimer's literature.

References

1   Rao T. Will fish sauce and charred oranges return the world Covid took from me? *The New York Times* 2021. www.nytimes.com/2021/03/02/dining/covid-loss-of-smell.html?referringSource=articleShare. (open access).

2   Hawkes, CH. Smell, taste and COVID-19: Testing is essential. *QJM: Int J Med* 2021; 114: 83–91. https://doi.org/10.1093/qjmed/hcaa326 (open access).

3   Wang L, Davis P, Volkow ND, *et al.* Association of COVID-19 with new-onset Alzheimer's disease. *J Alzheimers Dis* 2022; 89: 411–414. https://doi.org/10.3233/JAD-220717 (open access).

13 ALZHEIMER'S DISEASE AND WORK

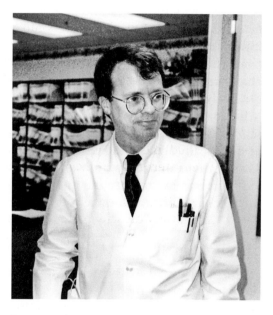

This photo from 1991 is, I believe, the only picture of me while working, long before gray hair and Alzheimer's – photo by Lois Seed.

Wendy Mitchell, in her extraordinary book, *Somebody I Used to Know: A Memoir*, tells of her frustration when asking her supervisors in the UK National Health Service to accommodate for her early-onset Alzheimer's disease [1]. Wendy herself was a supervisor, but with her MCI she was having trouble using a new database program. Otherwise, she was still able to do her job. Her supervisors were flummoxed and sent her to the Occupational Health department. As she walked into her appointment there, she saw the Occupational Health adviser reading online about What is Alzheimer's Disease? The only suggestion was early retirement. Wendy felt that with some accommodation, she would be able to work successfully for a while longer. When she told her own staff about her problem, they all pitched in to problem solve, making it possible for her to continue working.

The intersection of work and Alzheimer's can be fraught with misunderstanding, ignorance, and fear. Recall that Alzheimer's disease is a continuum. At one extreme is dementia. At the other extreme is preclinical Alzheimer's disease, with early deposition of amyloid plaques and neurofibrillary tangles in the brain, decades before any symptoms occur. Somewhere in the middle is MCI, which as the name suggests, is mild memory loss or other cognitive issues that do not yet interfere with daily activities including work.

Many people can continue to work with MCI and sometimes even with dementia. This will depend on the requirements of the job, and the worker with cognitive impairment may need to be accommodated to succeed. Remarkably, there has been relatively little research on this topic [2].

Workers with MCI or dementia are protected in the US by the Americans with Disabilities Act, although this protection may be limited by the severity of the cognitive impairment. Some possible accommodation tactics suggested by the Job Accommodation Network [3], under contract to the US Office of Disability Employment Policy, are listed by specific work problems. For executive function deficits (trouble making plans, easy distractibility), recommendations include using calendars and planners, checklists, color-coded systems, soundproof panels, flexible work schedules, job coaches, and/or written instructions. For time management issues, consider electronic organizers, timers and watches, reminders, personal on-site pagers, task separation, and/or written instructions. For memory issues, consider additional training time and training refreshers, apps for memory, a support person, recorded directives, messages, and materials, and/or color-coded manuals, outlines, and maps.

Clearly, the accommodations suggested above are meant to be tailored to an individual's unique situation. As a personal example, I retired before I had any measurable cognitive impairment because I knew I was on the Alzheimer's trajectory, and I wasn't going to take the chance of harming a patient because of a cognitive slip up. During the year following retirement, I volunteered at a free clinic providing general medical care under the supervision of an experienced specialist in internal or family medicine. As time went on, I stopped seeing patients altogether, and I did not renew my medical license, but my fund of neurological knowledge was still robust, so I was able to continue volunteer teaching on annual trips to Africa for another three years. Continued work will be possible for some, but it will probably require evolving the job into one with more supervision, perhaps less stress, and by building on the strengths that remain.

References

1   Mitchell W. *Somebody I Used to Know: A Memoir*. New York: Ballantine Books, 2018.
2   Silvaggi F, Leonardi M, Tiraboschi P, *et al*. Keeping people with dementia or mild cognitive impairment in employment: A literature review on its determinants. *Int J Environ Res Public Health* 2020; 17: 842. https://doi.org/10.3390/ijerph17030842 (open access).

3   Job Accommodation Network. Accommodation and
    Compliance Series: Employees with Alzheimer's
    Disease. 2022. https://askjan.org/disabilities/Alzheimer-
    s-Disease.cfm accessed November 16, 2022 (open
    access).

14 CROSSWORD CONTROVERSIES

Over and over, perhaps *ad nauseum*, I have been talking about the evidence-based lifestyle changes that can reduce the risk of getting Alzheimer's disease and/or slow its progression. These include getting frequent aerobic exercise, eating a Mediterranean-style diet, staying intellectually and socially engaged, getting adequate (but not too much sleep), and controlling cardiovascular risk factors including diabetes, high blood pressure, high cholesterol, smoking, and obesity. All of these measures are most effective if started in or before middle age and have much less value if started after the onset of cognitive impairment.

Let's concentrate here on intellectual activity. There is clear evidence that life-long learning builds cognitive reserve and delays the onset of cognitive loss without much if any slowing of the progression of the amyloid plaques and neurofibrillary tangles. Intellectual activity appears to make the brain more resilient to the neuropathological ravages of Alzheimer's. It helps build cognitive reserve. What about doing brain games and crossword puzzles? The evidence has been conflicting over the years. One paper from 2014 showed that subjects who did crossword puzzles were 2.54 years slower to begin cognitive impairment than those who didn't do crosswords [1]. At autopsy, there was no difference in the two groups in number of plaques and tangles. The brains looked the same, but those who did crosswords had a slower trajectory until near the end when they appeared to catch up with the non-puzzlers.

Most recent studies have shown little if any benefit from doing crossword puzzles alone. To quote Lisa Genova from her book *Remember: The Science of Memory and the Art of Forgetting*:

> There is no compelling evidence that doing puzzles or brain-training exercises does anything to decrease your risk of Alzheimer's. You'll improve at doing crosswords, but you're not building a bigger, Alzheimer's resistant brain. You don't want to simply retrieve information you've already learned, because this type of mental exercise is like traveling down old, familiar streets. ... You want to pave new neural roads. Building an Alzheimer's-resistant brain through cognitive stimulation means learning to play the piano, meeting new friends, traveling to a new city, or reading this book [2].

As she says, it is more effective to build new brain pathways and synapses than to simply retrieve information stored in your memory.

However, a recent study gives crossword puzzle solving some unexpected support [3]. Subjects with MCI were randomized to spend 30 minutes, four times per week for 12 weeks doing either moderately difficult crossword puzzles, equivalent to the Thursday crossword in the *New York Times*, or computerized cognitive training games on the Luminosity platform. Over the course of the 78-week study, the subjects had six additional booster doses of crosswords or computer games. Surprisingly, the subjects doing crosswords had slower cognitive decline than those doing computer games. Also, MRI scans showed significantly less atrophy of the hippocampus, an important brain center for memory consolidation, in those doing crosswords compared to those doing computer games. A significant weakness of this study is that there was no control group, a group that did neither crosswords nor cognitive games.

Still, the results are provocative and unexpected, even by the authors of the study.

The potential benefit of doing brain exercises remains unsettled. Certainly, there is no harm in these activities. If you like to do crosswords as I do, then by all means keep doing them. I try to make it a learning exercise rather than just retrieving words from memory. Toward the end of the week when the clues get hard, I pause and look up that lake in Africa I have never heard of, or that inventor of the mechanical computer, Charles Babbage. I try to learn something new from every puzzle, and I suspect that is helping to sprout some new connections in my brain.

Whatever you do, keep on learning. Learn in ways that are enjoyable to you. Read new books, keep a journal, try learning a new language, try out new ideas on friends and family, and yes, if you like doing crossword puzzles, keep on doing them.

References

1   Pillai JA, Hall CB, Dickson DW, *et al.* Association of crossword puzzle participation with memory decline in persons who develop dementia. *J Int Neuropsychol Soc* 2011; 17(6): 1006–1013. https://doi.org/10.1017/S1355617711001111. PMID: 22040899; PMCID: PMC3885259 (open access).
2   Genova L. *Remember: The Science of Memory and the Art of Forgetting.* New York: Harmony Books, 2021, p. 224.
3   Devanand DP, Goldberg TE, Qian M, *et al.* Computerized games versus crosswords training in mild cognitive impairment. *NEJM Evid* 2022; 1(12). https://doi.org/10.1056/EVIDoa2200121.

15 CAN LONELINESS INCREASE RISK FOR DEMENTIA?

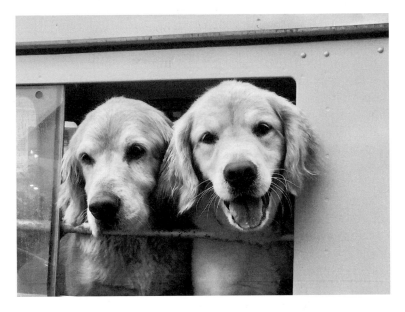

The antithesis of loneliness – best friends waiting outside a restaurant in Mystic, Connecticut, for their morning bacon treat.

Depression and loneliness are common among people with dementia, including Alzheimer's disease, and a recent paper in *Neurology* suggests that loneliness may actually increase the chance of getting dementia [1]. This was a retrospective analysis of data collected from the Framingham Study (September 9, 1948–December 31, 2018). At baseline, the 2,038 participants were dementia-free and had loneliness assessed using one question from a depression rating scale. They were asked how often they had felt lonely in the previous week. Participants were classified as lonely (3–7 days) or not lonely (0–2 days). Ten years later, those in the lonely group were 1½ times more likely to have dementia than those who were self-rated as not lonely at baseline. Also, among those who still did not have dementia at the 10-year mark, the participants who had self-rated as lonely were more likely to have poorer executive function (associated with prefrontal damage), smaller cerebral cortex volume, and more white matter brain damage despite scoring in the normal range on cognitive tests for dementia.

The results were interpreted as supporting the hypothesis that loneliness can be a driver of dementia pathology, increasing the risk of getting dementia. However, the authors admitted that there could be another explanation; loneliness could be an early symptom of dementia, perhaps occurring years before the onset of cognitive problems. They felt this was relatively unlikely given the 10-year hiatus between the onset of loneliness and the diagnosis of dementia.

I disagree. I think that both hypotheses are plausible, and perhaps both are correct, at least for Alzheimer's disease. The key here is understanding that Alzheimer's pathology in the brain, the amyloid plaques and neurofibrillary tangles, can start to form up to 20 years before there is any cognitive impairment. Loss of the ability to smell is almost universal in Alzheimer's, and it often begins years before the cognitive impairment. In fact, Alzheimer's pathology is first seen in olfactory centers in the brain, later followed by the hippocampus and other memory-processing areas. The prefrontal cortex is also an early site of beta-amyloid deposition. This area of the brain is involved in executive function; making plans and decisions, expressing personality, and moderating social behavior.

Damage to the prefrontal cortex often results in apathy, an early symptom of Alzheimer's disease. As an example, the amyloid PET scan of my brain done as part of a research study in 2015 shows moderate amounts of amyloid in my prefrontal cortex as well as in two olfactory centers, the piriform cortex and the mesial orbitofrontal cortex. At that time, my cognitive testing was still in the normal range, but I had started to lose my sense of smell almost ten years before, and my abilities to make plans and socialize were already affected.

My point is this. Loss of the sense of smell is an early, nonspecific symptom of Alzheimer's disease. It can start many years before there is any cognitive impairment. Amyloid deposition in the prefrontal cortex can also cause early personality changes including apathy before there is any cognitive change. I think it is entirely possible that loneliness may be another early, nonspecific symptom of Alzheimer's. Perhaps loneliness might also predispose to getting dementia as proposed in this paper. We don't know the answer yet.

Why is this important? It is becoming increasingly apparent that our first success with treating Alzheimer's disease will come in the earliest stages, before cognitive impairment and death of nerve cells in the brain have progressed. Identifying these people who are on the Alzheimer's trajectory but who do not yet have cognitive problems will be difficult. It may be possible to combine some of these nonspecific, pre-cognitive impairment symptoms, loss of smell, personality and apathy issues, with family history risks and known genetic markers to identify those who might benefit from more precise testing with blood biomarkers or PET scans. Early identification of Alzheimer's disease before cognitive impairment has started is controversial, but it may be necessary for successful treatment.

References

1   Salinas J, Beiser AS, Samra JK, *et al*. Association of loneliness with 10-year dementia risk and early markers of vulnerability for neurocognitive decline. *Neurology* 2022; 98: e1337–e1348. https://doi.org/10.1212/WNL.000000000020 0039 (open access).

16 EXCESSIVE LAXATIVE USE AND DEMENTIA

My mother was an avid book collector. As a teen, I would browse the bookshelves in our home looking for interesting nuggets. One of my favorite finds was *The Importance of Living* by the Chinese philosopher Lin Yutang. The book was originally published in 1937, but I am not certain when the copy in our home was published.

At my small high school in the 1960s, we had a meeting every morning for announcements by the faculty and inspirational readings by students on the "chapel" committee. When my turn came to read, it was often an excerpt from *The Importance of Living*. The only adage I remember now is "If one's bowels move, one is happy, and if they don't move, one is unhappy. That is all there is to it." At the time I shared this wisdom with the school, I was probably trying to be cheeky if not downright scatological, but I have realized over the years that there is some truth to that aphorism. On the dark side, an obsession with regular bowel movements can encourage an overuse of laxatives leading to unintended consequences.

The term "gut microbiota" refers to the various organisms normally living symbiotically in our intestines. These bacteria, viruses, fungi, and yeasts start to colonize the gut at birth, and reach a stable population at about age three. The health of the gut microbiota is essential for our own health. Throughout life, excessive use of some antibiotics and laxatives can disrupt the composition of the gut microbiota leading to problems not only in the gut but also throughout the body, including the brain [1].

A recent study in *Neurology* provides the best data yet on the effect of long-term, chronic laxative use on the risk of getting dementia [2]. In this 10-year study of 502,229 UK Biobank participants, the regular use of laxatives was associated with higher risk of all-cause and vascular dementia. At the start of the study, the average age was 57 years, and none of the participants had dementia. Over the subsequent 10 years, 1.3% of those who regularly used laxatives developed dementia. Regular use was defined as taken almost every day. Only 0.4% of those not regularly using laxatives developed dementia. After adjusting for factors such as age, sex, education, other illnesses, and medication use, participants who regularly used laxatives were 1.51 times more likely to develop dementia compared to people who did not regularly use laxatives (hazard ratio = 1.51). The risk of dementia also increased with the number of laxative types used at the same time. For people using one type of laxative, the hazard ratio was 1.28 compared to 1.90 for people taking two or more types of laxatives. Osmotic laxatives (e.g., polyethylene glycol, milk of magnesia, or lactulose) were the worst offenders when used regularly, even when taken individually. The authors concluded that "instead of regular use of laxatives, constipation can be mitigated most of the time by lifestyle changes, such as increasing fluid intake, dietary fiber, and activity levels, which may also benefit brain health." Lin Yutang might well have approved of such advice.

References

1   Rutsch A, Kantsjö JB, Ronchi F. The gut-brain axis: How microbiota and host inflammasome influence brain physiology and pathology. *Front Immunol* 2020;

11: 604179. https://doi.org/10.3389/fimmu.2020.604179. PMID: 33362788; PMCID: PMC7758428 (open access).

2　Yang Z, Wei C, Li X, *et al.* Association between regular laxative use and incident dementia in UK Biobank participants. *Neurology* 2023; 100: e1702–e1711. https://doi.org/10.1212/WNL.0000000000 207081.

17 DOG DEMENTIA (CANINE COGNITIVE DYSFUNCTION)

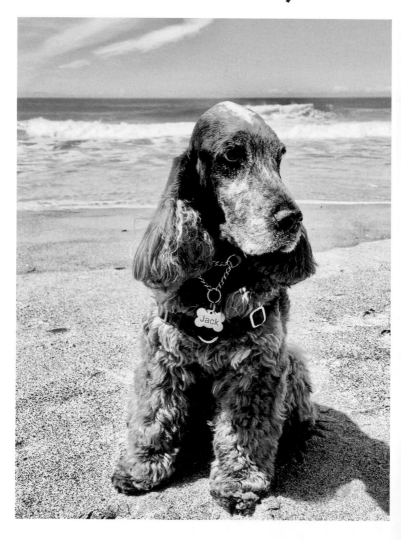

Jack, our English cocker spaniel, is eight years old, middle-aged for a dog. He may be a little neurotic, after all he is a spaniel, but he is still sharp as a tack and has no signs yet of cognitive impairment. It turns out that many mammals do develop cognitive impairment toward the end of their lives. In dogs, this cognitive decline is called canine cognitive dysfunction (CCD), and it occurs in up to 60% of dogs over 11 years of age. It is more common in small dogs, probably because they tend to live longer than large dogs. As we shall see, it has similarities, and some differences, compared to Alzheimer's disease in humans [1].

What does dementia look like in dogs? Obviously, the type of cognitive tests done in humans are, for the most part, impossible to use with dogs. The clues to CCD are changes in behavior. The acronym DISHAA (Disorientation, altered social Interactions, altered Sleep–wake cycles, House soiling and loss of other learned behaviors, altered Activity levels, and increasing Anxiety) has been proposed as a guide for assessment. A dog with dementia might simply stare into space for long periods of time. He might sleep during the day and be active at night. He might be unwilling to interact with other pets or even his people. The ability to smell is often decreased, just as it is in humans with Alzheimer's disease. Several veterinary tests have been developed to grade dog cognition such as the Canine Cognitive Dysfunction Rating Scale (CCDR) comprised of 13 behavioral items evaluating orientation, memory, apathy, impaired olfaction, and locomotion [2].

Although age-related cognitive dysfunction has been reported in a number of elderly mammals including cats, horses, apes, bears, dolphins, and most species of non-human primates, most investigations have been done on dogs. The brain pathology in all of these species is very similar to that found in Alzheimer's disease in humans. Beta-amyloid plaques are found outside of nerve cells in more or less the same parts of the brain across species. Beta-amyloid is also found in the walls of small blood vessels in the brains of humans with Alzheimer's as well as in most of these animals. This so-called cerebral amyloid angiopathy is an important cause of brain hemorrhages in elderly humans, and it has been reported to be a cause of brain bleeding in elderly dogs as well. Abnormal phosphorylated tau protein has been found in dogs, but unlike in humans, it does not seem to form into neurofibrillary tangles. Perhaps non-human animals do not live long enough for tangles to develop. Interestingly, mice and rats do not develop dementia. At least normal, unmanipulated rodents don't get it. Are you puzzled? Transgenic mice have been the mainstay of building animal models of Alzheimer's disease. In a transgenic mouse, human genes for Alzheimer's are inserted into the mouse genome and then the mice are bred into a new strain that regularly gets an Alzheimer's-like disease. These transgenic mice have been very important models for testing theories and possible interventions for Alzheimer's disease. But normal, wild-type mice do not get dementia.

What can be done for a dog with dementia? Is it an unavoidable part of aging? Probably not. Just as some humans live into their 90s without getting Alzheimer's or other dementias, not all elderly dogs develop CCD. Recent studies have shown that the risk of a dog developing cognitive dysfunction is inversely associated with the amount of daily activity. The greater the daily activity throughout life, the lower the chance of a dog developing CCD as he ages [3]. Prevention may be the key, just as in humans. For dogs that do develop CCD, the vet may recommend a special diet, structured activity including regular walks, good daytime sunlight to help maintain a proper sleep cycle, and careful use of certain antidepressants for anxiety. Some studies have found cognitive improvement from cholinesterase inhibitors such as donepezil (Aricept) [4,5], but benefits are subtle and side effects can be an issue. It is generally best to avoid the use of medications except under the expert guidance of a veterinarian.

References

1 Prpar Mihevc S, Majdic G. Canine cognitive dysfunction and Alzheimer's disease – Two facets of the same disease? *Front Neurosci* 2019; 13: 604. https://doi.org/10.3389/fnins.2019.00604 (open access).

2 Salvin HE, McGreevy PD, Sachdev PS, Valenzuela MJ. The canine cognitive dysfunction rating scale (CCDR): A data-driven and ecologically relevant assessment tool. *Vet J* 2011; 188: 331–336. https://doi.org/10.1016/j.tvjl.2010.05.014 (open access).

3 Bray EE, Raichlen DA, Forsyth KK, *et al.* Dog Aging Project Consortium. Associations between physical activity and cognitive dysfunction in older companion dogs: Results from the Dog Aging Project. *Geroscience* 2023; 45: 645–661. https://doi.org/10.1007/s11357-022-00655-8; Epub 2022 Sep 21; PMID: 36129565; PMCID: PMC9886770 (open access).

4 Zakošek Pipan M, Prpar Mihevc S, Štrbenc M, *et al.* Treatment of canine cognitive dysfunction with novel butyrylcholinesterase inhibitor. *Sci Rep* 2021; 11: 18098. https://doi.org/10.1038/s41598-021-97404-2 (open access).

5 Araujo JA, Greig NH, Ingram DK, Sandin J, de Rivera C, Milgram NW. Cholinesterase inhibitors improve both memory and complex learning in aged beagle dogs. *J Alzheimers Dis* 2011; 26: 143–155. https://doi.org/10.3233/JAD-2011-110005. PMID: 21593569; PMCID: PMC4979003 (open access).

18 THE POSSIBLE ROLE OF BRAIN INFLAMMATION IN ALZHEIMER'S DISEASE MAY BE MORE SIGNIFICANT IN APOE-4 CARRIERS

I'm almost 72 years old, and it is still hard for me to believe I'm not 40 anymore like my son Adam. I think the attack of Alzheimer's on my memories has speeded up time for me. Where did it all go? But I am starting to get some reminders of my true age thanks to arthritis in my fingers and other joints. Inflammation is a source of pain and joint destruction as we age, and the pharmaceutical industry is happy to supply us with anti-inflammatory medications to ease our discomfort. Inflammation not only affects our joints. It can cause problems throughout our bodies.

For over 20 years, there has been growing evidence of the importance of inflammation in Alzheimer's disease [1]. Briefly, there have been a number of observations that people taking anti-inflammatory medications, particularly those with rheumatoid arthritis, may have a modestly reduced risk of getting Alzheimer's disease. Studies in animal models have shown that brain inflammation has a dual response, protective in the acute reaction and detrimental when chronic. In these animal studies, chronic neuroinflammation activates inflammatory cells in the brain called microglia, increases beta-amyloid burden, and increases the production of hyperphosphorylated tau, the toxic form of tau protein found in neurofibrillary tangles. However, trials of anti-inflammatory medications such as ibuprofen in humans have for the most part failed to show a significant reduction in risk of getting Alzheimer's. Recent work has suggested that this damaging effect of inflammation on Alzheimer's risk does indeed occur in humans but is specific to those carrying the *APOE-4* allele [2].

This is one more example of the heterogeneity of Alzheimer's disease. Alzheimer's disease associated with *APOE-4* appears to be a different disease than Alzheimer's disease in the absence *APOE-4*. I think this is an important reason why it has been so hard to find an effective medication to treat Alzheimer's. Anti-amyloid monoclonal antibodies such as aducanumab and lecanemab also appear to be more effective in patients with *APOE-4*-associated Alzheimer's disease compared to those who are not *APOE-4* carriers [3]. I am hopeful that as we learn more about the genetic and biochemical differences in these diseases that we have lumped together as Alzheimer's, we will finally be able to develop targeted therapies for all of these variants.

References

1   Kinney JW, Bemiller SM, Murtishaw AS, Leisgang AM, *et al.* Inflammation as a central mechanism in Alzheimer's disease. *Alzheimers Dement* 2018; 4: 575–590. https://doi.org/10.1016/j.trci.2018.06.014. PMID: 30406177; PMCID: PMC6214864 (open access).

2   Tao Q, Fang Ang TFAA, Akhter-Khan SC, *et al.* Impact of
    C-reactive protein on cognition and Alzheimer disease
    biomarkers in homozygous *APOE ε4* carriers. *Neurology*
    2021; 97: e1243–e1252. https://doi.org/10.1212/WNL.00
    00000000012512.
3   Swanson CJ, Zhang Y, Dhadda S, *et al.* A randomized,
    double-blind, phase 2b proof-of-concept clinical trial in
    early Alzheimer's disease with lecanemab, an anti-Aβ
    protofibril antibody. *Alz Res Therapy* 2021; 13: 80. https://
    doi.org/10.1186/s13195-021-00813-8 (open access).

19 SURPRISINGLY GOOD NEWS ABOUT THE ACETYLCHOLINESTERASE INHIBITORS (DONEPEZIL, RIVASTIGMINE, AND GALANTAMINE)

When I finished my training and started practicing neurology in 1989, there were absolutely no medications that mitigated cognitive deterioration in patients with Alzheimer's disease. There were drugs for some of the unwanted symptoms such as sleep reversal, depression, anger outbursts, and seizures, but nothing to address the underlying progressive brain damage leading to cognitive impairment, dementia, and ultimately death. I remember feeling very frustrated that I could offer nothing at all, not even hope. Then, in 1993, the first acetylcholinesterase inhibitor (AChEI), tacrine, was approved by the FDA for treatment of dementia. This class of medication is thought to work by raising levels of acetylcholine, an important neurotransmitter in the brain. There was a lot of excitement about the approval of tacrine, but almost immediately severe side effects including serious liver damage were encountered, and the use of the drug dwindled and disappeared almost overnight. I don't think I ever wrote a prescription for tacrine. Three years later, the first relatively safe AChEI, donepezil (trade name Aricept), was approved and it is still going strong. Within a few years, two similar drugs, rivastigmine and galantamine, were approved. They all were about equally effective. They all had similar side effects, but sometimes a person could tolerate one better than another. For an individual patient, it was hard to tell for sure if it was effective or not. A few of my patients had remarkable improvement and others didn't seem to change much at all. For others, the side effects were intolerable. Most common were nausea, cramps, and diarrhea as well as nightmares and insomnia. I found that starting my patients at a very low dose, lower than recommended, and very slowly increasing the dose over several months would usually avoid the side effects.

When I started taking donepezil myself a few years ago, I went through the usual gastrointestinal (GI) upset, but what bothered me most were terrible nightmares almost every night. I asked my neurologist and learned that nightmares are common and can usually be avoided by taking the daily dose in the morning, not at bedtime. Sure enough, that did the trick. Now I have no side effects at all. But is it helping me? Hard to know. At times I think it has helped, but the placebo effect may be responsible for that. Information from one patient's experience is really of no use in evaluating a treatment despite what you hear every night from the plethora of TV endorsements for memory enhancing products. What is needed is a large, carefully controlled clinical trial. Most of the small trials in the past showed a modest slowing of cognitive impairment for a few years but little if any benefit in the severe dementia stage. No one had claimed that this class of medications could allow people with Alzheimer's disease to live longer.

Recently, a paper in *Scientific Reports* described an observational study to evaluate the rate of cognitive decline, as well as the overall survival, in a large sample of patients affected by dementia, treated or not treated with AChEIs, in a real-world setting [1]. The data were retrieved from a large database, the National Alzheimer's Coordinating Center Uniform Data Set, and included 4,032 subjects with Alzheimer's disease, Lewy body disease, and vascular dementia. Subjects were carefully matched to eliminate confounding differences leaving 786 who had received AChEIs and 786 who had not. Cognitive status was assessed with the Mini-Mental Status Exam (MMSE). The results were remarkable. First, subjects with Lewy body disease had no cognitive benefit from treatment. However, those with Alzheimer's disease who received an AChEI had almost no change in the MMSE score for six years while subjects not taking an AChEI continued to decline. This is important to understand. The people receiving an AChEI did not have improved cognition, the metric I had used to judge success, but they did not get worse for about six years. At the end of follow up in year 12, subjects with Alzheimer's taking an AChEI had an average 5.7-point decrease in MMSE score from onset compared to those not taking an AChEI who decreased an average of 10.8 points. Keep in mind that the top score on the MMSE is 30 and the cutoff for dementia is 23 and below [2], so the AChEI treated subjects had, on average, remained above the dementia cutoff until near the end of the study.

The same pattern although not as pronounced was seen in subjects with vascular dementia. I suspect this reflects the high incidence of comorbidity. Nearly a third of dementia brains seen at autopsy have both Alzheimer's and vascular dementia pathology [3].

In addition to the slowing of cognitive decline, there was a strong association between AChEI therapy and lower all-cause mortality. This was true even for subjects with Lewy body disease who had no cognitive benefit from taking AChEI drugs. This suggests to me that the increased survival associated with these drugs must have a different mechanism than that resisting cognitive decline.

Very similar mortality results were reported almost simultaneously in a meta-analysis of 24 studies reporting mortality in dementia patients taking AChEI drugs [4]. Treatment with these medications was associated with significantly lower all-cause mortality (adjusted hazard ratio 0.77). In other words, patients with dementia treated with drugs such as donepezil were 23% less likely to die over time than those not taking these drugs.

These papers have forced me to change my opinion of AChEIs in the treatment of Alzheimer's disease. As a neurologist I was skeptical that they had much benefit, but because they were relatively safe to take, I routinely prescribed them. For those patients of mine who struggled with side effects, I would have a low threshold for stopping the drug. Now, if I were still seeing patients with Alzheimer's disease or vascular dementia, I would strongly encourage persisting with the drug, starting out at very low doses if necessary, and increasing the dose very slowly as tolerated and needed. The benefit seems to be real, even in the later stages of the disease.

References

1   Zuin M, Cherubini A, Volpato, S, *et al.* Acetyl-cholines-terase-inhibitors slow cognitive decline and decrease overall mortality in older patients with dementia. *Sci Rep* 2022; **12**: 12214. https://doi.org/10.1038/s41598-022-16476-w (open access).

2   O'Bryant SE, Humphreys JD, Smith GE, *et al.* Detecting dementia with the Mini-Mental State Examination in highly educated individuals. *Arch Neurol* 2008; 65: 963–967.   https://doi.org/10.1001/archneur.65.7.963 (open access).

3   Rabinovici GD, Carrillo MC, Forman M, *et al.* Multiple comorbid neuropathologies in the setting of Alzheimer's disease neuropathology and implications for drug development. *Alzheimers Dement: Transl Res Clin Interv* 2017; 3: 83–91. https://doi.org/10.1016/j.trci.2016.09.002 (open access).

4   Truong C, Recto C, Lafont C, *et al*. Effect of cholinester-
    ase inhibitors on mortality in patients with dementia: a
    systematic review of randomized and nonrandomized
    trials. *Neurology* 2022; 99: e2313–e2325. https://doi.org/
    10.1212/WNL.0000000000201161.

20 MORE ABOUT THE IMPORTANCE OF EXERCISE

Due to a series of unforeseen events this week, both of our children living in Portland needed additional help caring for their children, four of our five grandchildren. There is nothing I like better than spending time with my grandchildren, but instead of seeing them a few times each week, we have suddenly been spending a lot of time with one or both sets every day. It's been great, but what I have missed out on is my daily 10,000 steps of aerobic exercise. I have been lucky on some of these days to get 4,000 steps. And I can feel the result. All week I have been more befuddled than usual. Some of this is doubtless due to the change in schedule, but I think much if not most of my increased confusion has been caused by decreased exercise.

Today, we have no childcare responsibilities. It is a beautiful, sunny day in Portland, and Jack and I have already covered 10,566 steps, 4.25 miles, and a total elevation gain of 633 feet in two walks this morning. I'm feeling really good. My smartphone cognitive test score just now is 8% better than my average score.

Aerobic exercise is good for the brain. If started in midlife it can reduce the chance of getting Alzheimer's disease by up to 50% [1]. I don't think the mechanism for this long-term benefit is fully understood, but it probably is due to a combination of increasing blood flow to the brain, altering the release of certain stress hormones, moderating inflammation, improving cardiovascular health, and reducing the occurrence of small strokes [2]. There is also a well-documented acute effect of exercise [3]. Again, the cause is not well understood and has generally been attributed to increased brain blood flow while exercising. For me, this cognitive boost lasts for at least several hours after completing a workout.

A very interesting recent study in older people (average age 65 years) who did not have dementia or MCI suggests a novel mechanism that may play a role in the beneficial cognitive effects of exercise. Half of the subjects underwent a 20-week dance-based aerobic exercise program that met for 60 minutes twice weekly [4]. The other half carried on as usual with no special intervention. Both groups were assessed using a functional MRI (fMRI) method designed to measure the flexibility of neuronal networks, particularly within the medial temporal lobe (MTL), a part of the brain that is home to the hippocampus and is key to learning and memory. At the end of the 20 weeks, the subjects who underwent the exercise regimen had a significant increase in the flexibility of this MTL network, suggesting that even in this short period of time there had been an improvement in function of this important network involved in learning and consolidation of memory. The take home point is that exercise improves the flexibility and efficiency of an important neuronal network thought to be involved in learning and memory, at least in these older subjects who are still cognitively normal. This has not yet been studied in people who are already cognitively impaired by dementia.

The beneficial effects of exercise on memory are real, and there appear to be several mechanisms involved. Exercise reduces the risk of getting Alzheimer's, and it slows the progression once it has begun. Exercise also acutely improves cognitive function both in normal people and in those with MCI. The time to start a regular aerobic exercise program is in midlife, not after dementia has taken hold. I can't stress this enough; exercise is probably the most effective tool we now have for the prevention and slowing of Alzheimer's disease.

References

1   Buchman AS, Boyle PA, Yu L, *et al.* Total daily physical activity and the risk of AD and cognitive decline in older adults. *Neurology* 2012; 78: 1323–1329. https://doi.org/10.1212/WNL.0b013e3182535d35; PMID: 22517108; PMCID: PMC3335448 (open access version).

2   Elsworthy RJ, Dunleavy C, Whitham M, *et al.* Exercise for the prevention of Alzheimer's disease: Multiple pathways to promote non-amyloidogenic AβPP processing. *Aging Health Res* 2022; 2: 100093. https://doi.org/10.1016/j.ahr.2022.100093 (open access).

3   Chang YK, Labban JD, Gapin JI, *et al.* The effect of acute exercise on cognitive performance: A meta-analysis. *Brain Res* 2012; 1453: 87–101. https://doi.org/10.1016/j.brainres.2012.02.068.

4   Sinha N, Berg CN, Yassa MA, *et al.* Increased dynamic flexibility in the medial temporal lobe network following an exercise intervention mediates generalization of prior learning. *Neurobiol Learn Mem* 2021; 177: 107340. https://doi.org/10.1016/j.nlm.2020.107340.

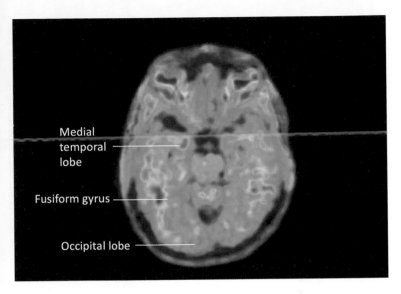

This is my 2018 tau-PET scan (done for a research study) showing abnormal tau protein (red and yellow colors) extending from the medial temporal lobes posteriorly into the region of the fusiform gyrus. Courtesy of Dr. Gil Rabinovici, UCSF Memory and Aging Center.

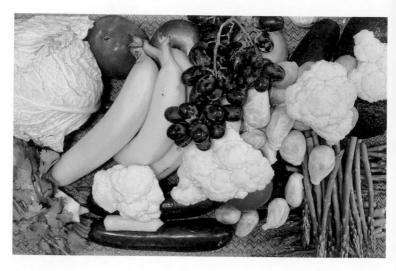

Healthy produce

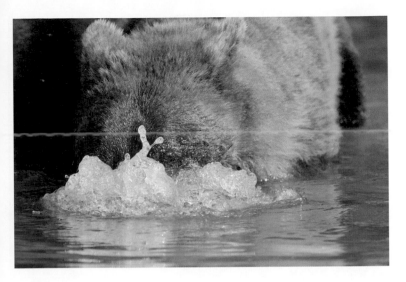

A Kodiak bear fishing for clams in Alaska.

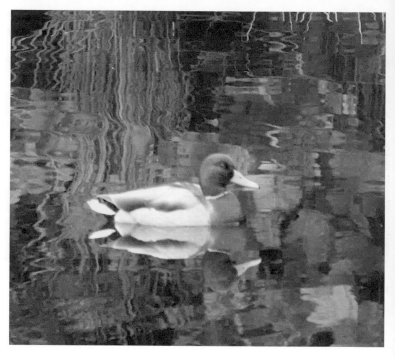

In the style of Monet.

Moonrise over Portland. The blurry lights on the US Bank Tower are on the left.

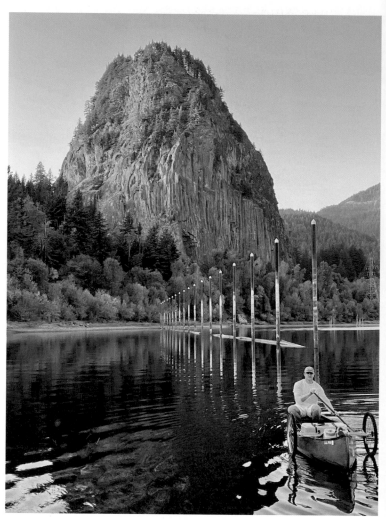

John Kraft in his canoe with Beacon Rock in the background. The bicycle wheels are used for portaging around dams.

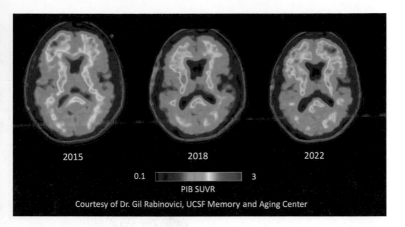

2015   2018   2022

0.1   3

PIB SUVR

Courtesy of Dr. Gil Rabinovici, UCSF Memory and Aging Center

These are amyloid PET scans of my brain in 2015, 2018, and 2022. Beta-amyloid shows up as yellow, orange, and red depending on the amount in that area. These are horizontal slices through my brain at a level just above the eyes.

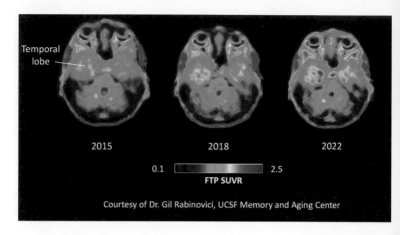

Courtesy of Dr. Gil Rabinovici, UCSF Memory and Aging Center

These are tau PET scans of my brain at the level of the eyes and anterior temporal lobes. Yellow, orange, and red represent increasing concentrations of tau. The intense red in the eyes is off-target labeling that appears in normal people as well.

21 ROLLING ON THE RIVER

Over the last 15 years I have taken many trips through the Columbia River Gorge on my mini-tugboat, *Lizzie G.* In the Pacific Northwest and perhaps elsewhere there used to be a tradition of naming commercial tugboats for the patriarchs and matriarchs of the boat owner's family. *Lizzie G* is named for my mother, Elizabeth Gibbs, although the only person who called her Lizzie was my father. My parents would be 112 and 114 today if still alive, but I think of them both when I am on the boat. My father loved boats – my mother not so much.

The Columbia River originates in the mountains of British Columbia, runs north for a while, then south, then passes through an 80-mile-long, 4,000 ft deep gap in the Cascade Mountain Range called the Columbia River Gorge, and finally reaches the Pacific Ocean at Astoria, Oregon, 1,243 miles from its origin in Canada. Indigenous people have lived along the river with its abundance of salmon for at least 15,000 years. European mariners explored the outlet of the Columbia in the late eighteenth century, and in 1792, American Robert Gray captained the first non-indigenous boat to cross the treacherous bar at the mouth of the river and explore 13 miles upstream. The Lewis and Clark overland expedition (1803–1805) crossed the Rocky Mountains, canoed down the Snake River, the largest tributary of the Columbia, and continued down the Columbia to the Pacific Ocean. Both the Americans and British rapidly recognized the potential for extracting great wealth from the river and the surrounding lands from fur trapping. As the supply of beavers, muskrats, otters, and other furry animals decreased by the 1850s from overhunting, lumber and salmon became central to the economy of the Oregon Territory. The Columbia River played a key role in transporting these goods to be loaded onto ships in Portland and Astoria, and shipped all over the world.

The Columbia River still plays a central part in the commerce of the Northwest. In 2020, hydropower generated by multiple dams along the Columbia and its tributaries supplied over 50% of the electricity consumed in Oregon. Barges carry grain from farms in eastern Oregon and Washington down the river to be loaded onto ships bound for Japan and elsewhere. Recently, I saw an odd barge headed upriver pushed by a large tug and pulled by a smaller one. At a distance of several miles, I just couldn't make out the nature of its cargo. Up close, I could see that the barge was carrying huge wind turbine blades heading to a wind farm in the east. Wind power is growing rapidly in Oregon and Washington, and already makes up at least 7% of regional power production.

The Columbia River Gorge is incredibly beautiful. It is a protected National Scenic Area, so new building is severely restricted. One of my favorite spots is Cape Horn. It is on the Washington side of the river and consists of towering basalt columns, some rising several hundred feet above the river. During the rainy season, there are many waterfalls. A 2,382-foot railroad tunnel runs through the rock. Although there is an overlook trail, the only way to really see the rock formation is from the water.

Rail lines run along the shores on both sides of the river. Trains pass by every 30–40 minutes. Perhaps the most controversial rail cargo is crude oil from the east shipped to refineries in the west. Derailments and spills have occurred including one that started a fire threatening the small town of Mosier, Oregon in 2016.

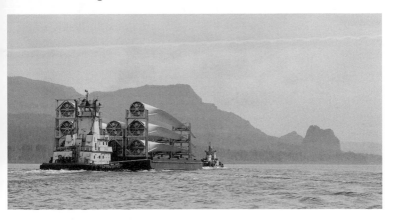

Wind turbine blades head to a wind farm in eastern Oregon or Washington.

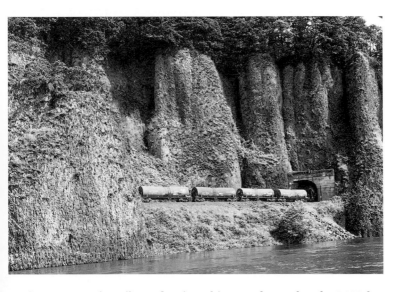

Tanker cars carrying oil to refineries. This tunnel stretches for 2,382 ft through the basalt rock of Cape Horn.

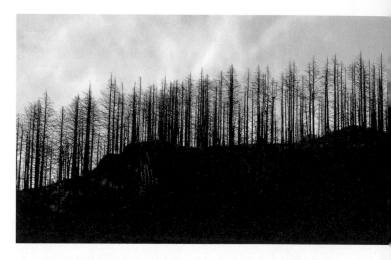

The scars of the 2017 Eagle Creek Fire as seen five years later.

Forest fires in the Columbia River Gorge are unfortunately becoming more common. In 2017, the Eagle Creek Fire burned for three months, eventually consuming 50,000 acres on the Oregon side of the Gorge. It was ignited by a teenager playing with fireworks.

The throbbing of a barge or rumble of a train will be heard frequently throughout the Gorge, but I don't find them to be intrusive. On a recent 1.9-mile hike to the top of Beacon Rock, 850 feet above the river below, I was surprised to hear an airplane. When I looked out, I was looking down, not up, at a plane below, banking hard to the right to circle around for a second view of the Rock. I am certain that this was the first and probably only time in my life that I could look down on a plane while standing on the ground!

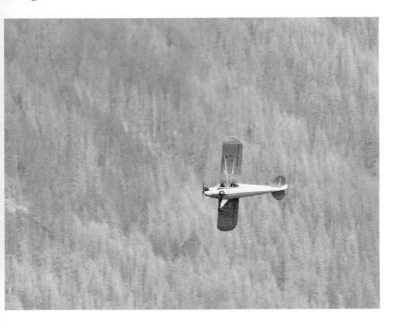

After descending from Beacon Rock, I took a breather on the dock at the base of the Rock, and I suddenly heard a whirring noise that I couldn't immediately identify. I looked up and there was a large drone hovering overhead. It was another first – the first drone I have seen or heard in the Gorge. Actually, drones are prohibited in many places in the Gorge over safety concerns, but perhaps the owner had not read the rules, and frankly, I must admit, it was pretty cool!

Roll on river. My soul is refreshed.

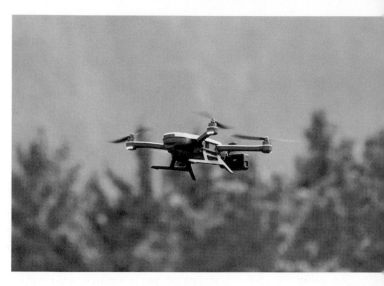

A drone hovers at the base of Beacon Rock.

22 THE MIND DIET REVISITED

Over the last 10 years or so, there have been an increasing number of studies that generally agree that people who regularly consume a plant-based, Mediterranean-style diet are less likely to get Alzheimer's dementia than those who do not. These studies have found nearly the same results in populations from around the world including the USA, Japan, Australia, Greece, and other European countries. The contents of the diets, age of participants, and extent of benefits may differ from study to study, but overall, those participants who follow a Mediterranean-style diet or one of the variants have between 35% and 50% less chance of getting Alzheimer's or, in some studies, all-cause dementia.

It has been tempting to sort out the parts of the Mediterranean diet that might be so beneficial in preventing dementia. The diet is rich in antioxidants, but trials of some of these antioxidants as supplements have been disappointing. A recent paper in *Neurology* suggests that the benefits of these antioxidants come from a complicated interaction with other nutrients in food. Trying to boost one potentially beneficial antioxidant as a supplement probably won't work. It seems that we need to get these good nutrients as part of the complete diet. No shortcuts allowed [1].

In 2015, the late Dr. Martha Clare Morris and her colleagues at Rush University published their first paper on the effects of following the MIND diet on the risk of getting Alzheimer's disease [2]. The Mediterranean-DASH Intervention for Neurodegenerative Delay (MIND) diet is a hybrid of the Mediterranean and Dietary Approaches to Stop Hypertension (DASH) diets, but it differs in the addition of berries and nuts, and stricter restrictions on dairy products. In that 2015 report, the MIND diet lowered the risk of developing Alzheimer's by as much as 53% in participants who adhered to the diet rigorously, and by about 35% in those who followed it only moderately well. These findings have been confirmed by several studies since then. In one head-to-head study, the MIND diet was more effective than the Mediterranean diet in preventing Alzheimer's [3]. The Rush group found that chemicals called flavonoids, and in particular a subgroup called flavonols, may be one of the keys to the success of the MIND and other Mediterranean-style diets. In a 2020 paper in *Neurology*, they showed that total flavonol consumption was inversely correlated with the chance of getting Alzheimer's disease [4]. Participants who ate the most flavonol-containing foods were less likely to get Alzheimer's as they aged compared to low flavonol consumers. The same group recently reported results of a prospective trial showing that higher dietary intakes of total flavonols and several individual flavonol constituents are associated with slower rates of decline in global cognition and multiple cognitive domains. These beneficial effects of flavonols on episodic memory, semantic memory, and visuospatial processing remained after adjusting for dietary intake of vitamin E, saturated fat, folate, lutein, and omega-3 fatty acids [5].

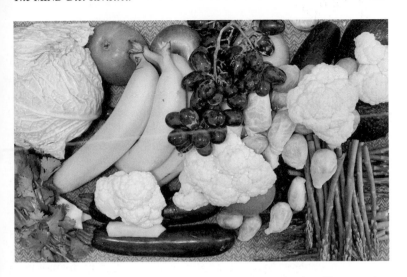

Healthy produce. (A black and white version of this figure will appear in some formats. For the color version, refer to the plate section.)

I had fun paging through the US Department of Agriculture (USDA) tables for flavonoid (and flavonol) content of various foods [6]. In general, the foods highest in total flavonols are various herbs, green vegetables (especially the bitter ones), and berries. By far the highest content in a vegetable of normal serving size is kale. Some of the herbs are higher on a per weight basis, but the serving size would be much less. Onions are a surprisingly good source of flavonols. At the bottom of the list, foods with undetectable flavonol levels, are avocados and mushrooms. Avocado oil has anti-inflammatory benefits of its own despite the absence of flavonol [7], so I will continue to enjoy my daily serving of avocado slices. Admittedly, kale may be an acquired taste, but it is part of my daily diet now, and I quite enjoy it both raw and cooked. Raw kale provides higher flavonol levels than when cooked.

Finally, there is increasing information suggesting that a flavonoid-rich diet can slow other degenerative diseases as well. A recent paper in the journal *Movement Disorders* found that adherence to either the MIND or Mediterranean diet delayed the onset of Parkinson's disease [8], and a paper in *Neurology* reported that adherence to the MIND diet decreased mortality in Parkinson's disease [9].

I have tried to adhere to the MIND diet as best I can. The main problem I have had was cheese. I love cheese, and I just couldn't limit myself to the recommended one serving per week. Then, last year, I discovered that I am lactose-intolerant. No more cheese or other dairy products. I do miss the cheese, but I can take solace in the fact that my adherence to the MIND diet is now 100%.

References

1   Beydoun MA, Beydoun HA, Fanelli-Kuczmarski MT, *et al.* Association of serum antioxidant vitamins and carotenoids with incident Alzheimer disease and all-cause dementia among US adults. *Neurology* 2022; 98: e2150–e2162. https://doi.org/10.1212/WNL.000000000200289.

2   Morris MC, Tangney CC, Wang Y, Sacks FM, Bennett DA, Aggarwal NT. MIND diet associated with reduced incidence of Alzheimer's disease. *Alzheimers Dement* 2015; 11: 1007–1014. https://doi.org/10.1016/j.jalz.2014.11.009. Epub 2015 Feb 11. PMID: 25681666; PMCID: PMC4532650 (open access).

3   Hosking DE, Eramudugolla R, Cherbuin N, *et al.* MIND not Mediterranean diet related to 12-year incidence of cognitive impairment in an Australian longitudinal cohort study. *Alzheimers Dement* 2019; 15: 581–589. https://doi.org/10.1016/j.jalz.2018.12.011.

4   Holland M, Agarwal P, Wang Y, *et al.* Dietary flavonols and risk of Alzheimer dementia. *Neurology* 2020; 94: e1749–e1756. https://doi.org/10.1212/WNL .0000000000008981.

5   Holland TM, Agarwal P, Wang Y, *et al.* Association of dietary intake of flavonols with changes in global cognition and several cognitive abilities. *Neurology* 2023; 100: e694–e702   https://doi.org/10.1212/WNL.000000000020 1541.

6   USDA Database for the Flavonoid Content of Selected Foods. Release 3.3 (March 2018). www.ars.usda.gov/ARSUserFiles/80400535/Data/Flav/Flav3.3.pdf   (open access) accessed March 15, 2023.

7   Flores M, Saravia C, Vergara CE, *et al.* Avocado oil: Characteristics, properties, and applications. *Molecules* 2019; 24: 2172. https://doi.org/10.3390/molecules2411 2172. PMID: 31185591; PMCID: PMC6600360 (open access).

8   Metcalfe-Roach A, Yu AC, Golz E, *et al.* MIND and Mediterranean diets associated with later onset of Parkinson's disease. *Movement Disorders* 2021; 36: 977–984. https://doi.org/10.1002/mds.28464 (open access).

9   Zhang X, Molsberry SA, Yeh T-A, *et al.* Intake of flavonoids and flavonoid-rich foods and mortality risk among individuals with Parkinson disease – A prospective cohort study. *Neurology* 2022; 98: e1064–e1076. https://doi.org/10.1212/WNL.0000000000 013275.

23 MY PHOTOGRAPHS, THEN AND NOW

In 1978, I was in the fifth year of the six-year Medical Scientist Training Program leading to MD and PhD degrees at Emory University in Atlanta, Georgia. It was a rigorous program, but I found time to also pursue my favorite hobby since childhood, photography. I took a series of advanced photography classes at the Callanwolde Community Arts Center, culminating in a course on the zone system. The zone system was developed by photographers Ansel Adams and Fred Archer in 1939–1940 as a way to focus attention on the shades of gray in a black and white photo through careful use of a spot light meter, a good eye for natural light, and sometimes, careful dodging and burning during exposure of the final print in the darkroom to lighten or darken areas of the image that might need tonal adjustment. Every print created with the zone system is unique.

That winter Lois and I discovered that flying from Atlanta to London for Christmas would be no more expensive than flying home to California to see our families as we usually did. I don't think my mother was particularly pleased with our decision, but we had a wonderful, Dickensian week in London complete with a blizzard on our final day. On Christmas morning, we walked across the street from our genteel-shabby hotel on Bayswater Road into Kensington Gardens and Hyde Park. The sun was just coming up and it was near freezing. Nobody else seemed to

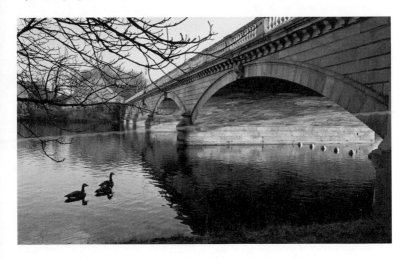

The Serpentine Bridge in Hyde Park, Christmas morning, 1978.

be up and about yet. As we came to the Serpentine Bridge, I was struck by the early morning light illuminating the underside of the bridge. As I got ready to take the shot, I saw geese approaching from the left, so I waited until they were silhouetted by the reflected sky before pressing the shutter release. It was just one shot on black and white film. When I returned to my darkroom in Atlanta, I darkened the tree branches in the left upper corner by selectively overexposing that portion of the print. This is one of my very favorite photographs. In fact, it won a prize in a photography contest in Atlanta in 1979, and the original silver print still hangs in our house.

Life got even busier in the 1980s with more clinical training, a research fellowship, a faculty appointment, more neurology training, and the birth of our three children. I didn't have time for working in the darkroom or taking long walks to find interesting things to photograph. Photography switched to a way of documenting

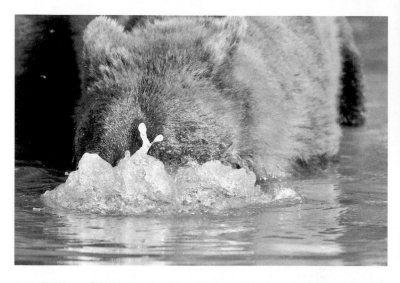

A Kodiak bear fishing for clams in Alaska. (A black and white version of this figure will appear in some formats. For the color version, refer to the plate section.)

our lives. I was unapologetically taking snapshots. In 2003, I made the switch to digital photography. I soon realized that I was no longer limited to a single or even a few attempts to get a good image. I could take as many as I wanted. It may have been sloppy, but it worked. After I retired in 2013, I once again had time to take photographs for the sake of creating a pleasing image, not just a documentation of life, although there is a lot of that too with five grandchildren keeping us wonderfully busy. I love to photograph birds and other wildlife, and the digital camera is perfect for this.

One of my favorite bird photos is this image of a mallard taken during a light breeze that rippled the water, creating a distortion that reminds me of Monet's impressionistic paintings from his garden in Giverny. It represents one more step in the evolution of my photography.

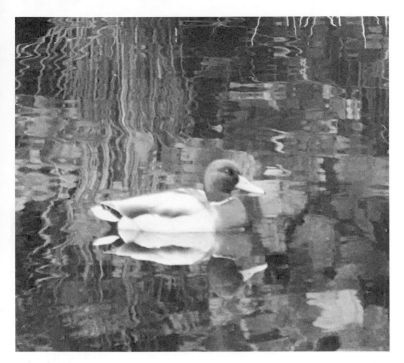

In the style of Monet. (A black and white version of this figure will appear in some formats. For the color version, refer to the plate section.)

As my Alzheimer's progresses, I now make more mistakes in adjusting the settings on my camera. I like to photograph the moon, especially when it is at its perigee, the closest distance to earth. On July 13, 2022, I took my camera, tripod, and telephoto lens down to an open lot several blocks away that allows a beautiful view of downtown Portland. I watched as the moon rose seemingly right next to the second tallest building in Portland, the US Bancorp Tower. I clicked away, rapidly capturing 20 or so images. None of the photos turned out well with one exception, and that one was a mistake. I had very limited visibility in the viewfinder due to the combination of darkness and my increasingly poor night vision. Given the strong contrast between the very bright moon and the trees in front of me, I did not realize that one of these images was shot through the branches of the tree. The automatic focus "thought" I was trying to photograph the trees, so these leaves are razor sharp, draped across the blurred image of the more distant moon and tall building. This photo is the antithesis of my structured, rule-following photograph of the Serpentine Bridge, but I quite like this somewhat ominous image. It might be a metaphor for my Alzheimer's-addled brain. Is it art? Is it any good? Does it really matter?

Moonrise over Portland. The blurry lights on the US Bank Tower are on the left. (A black and white version of this figure will appear in some formats. For the color version, refer to the plate section.)

24 DOES CATARACT SURGERY REALLY DECREASE THE RISK OF DEMENTIA?

Our vision appears to have a complicated relationship with dementia. Posterior cortical atrophy is a rare variant of Alzheimer's disease in which the amyloid plaques and neurofibrillary tangles first form in the back of the brain, in the visual cortex, and migrate toward the front of the brain, just the opposite of the more typical front to back progression in most Alzheimer's cases. The result is a progressive distortion and loss of vision sometimes progressing to blindness even before the onset of significant cognitive impairment. I have only seen one patient with posterior cortical atrophy. At first, I was sure she had a stroke or brain tumor, so I was completely surprised by her normal MRI, at least initially. I referred her to an expert who made the diagnosis of posterior cortical atrophy. In the subsequent months, she developed cognitive impairment leading eventually to dementia.

Subtle visual distortion is also fairly common in the more standard presentation of Alzheimer's. Visual-spatial perception can be altered, affecting one's ability to locate an object in space. The inability to recognize faces, prosopagnosia or face blindness, is common even early in Alzheimer's. In Lewy body dementia, very realistic visual hallucinations are common, often as the first sign of the disease.

But what about impaired vision? Does that have any effect on the risk of getting dementia? Several studies have suggested that it can, but the effect was felt to be relatively small. A recent paper in *JAMA Internal Medicine* suggests that the effect may be greater than we thought [1]. The study looked at over 3,000 subjects averaging 75 years of age who had a diagnosis of cataracts. Based on nearly 24,000 person-years of follow-up, cataract extraction was associated with a 29% reduced risk of getting dementia compared with participants with cataracts who did not have surgery. For a control group, people who had eye surgery for treatment of glaucoma had no change in their risk of dementia. The decreased risk of getting dementia after cataract surgery was attributed to the improvement in vision. Although no specific mechanism has been proposed, it seems possible to me that keeping the brain pathways for vision active may help preserve these visual processing centers in the brain, just as staying mentally active appears to have a protective effect in slowing the impairment of other cognitive functions. One caveat about interpreting this paper and most others I have seen about possible effects of visual loss on dementia risk is that the studies do not look at specific types of dementia. They are all lumped together. It is possible that the effects might be stronger for one dementia than another, say Alzheimer's *vs* frontotemporal dementia or Lewy body dementia. Still, it seems to be important to keep our senses as keen as possible along with the rest of our brain.

References

1   Lee CS, Gibbons LE, Lee AY, *et al.* Association between cataract extraction and development of dementia. *JAMA Intern Med* 2022; 182: 134–141. https://doi.org/10.1001/jamainternmed.2021.6990.

25 HEARING LOSS, APHASIA, AND DEMENTIA

Over the last 10 years or so, I have noticed increasing difficulty understanding what people are saying to me, especially if there are several people speaking at the same time, such as at a family dinner, or worse, at a big party. It may be the main reason why I find social occasions increasingly difficult and intimidating. When Lois speaks to me, I often have to ask her to repeat what she said. She has learned to say things twice if she wants me to get it. I know that is irritating for her. Often, I just nod or grunt, pretending I understand what she is saying. I have attributed this increasing problem to my Alzheimer's disease interfering with my ability to understand language, particularly if I don't hear every word clearly. Aphasias affecting language production (poor word finding) or reception (impaired understanding) are common in the mid-to-late stages of Alzheimer's, but trouble finding the right word or name is often one of the earliest symptoms of Alzheimer's.

In the last few months, I have noticed that Lois and I have markedly different choices for the volume when watching TV. She finds it is too loud when I set it, and I have to cup my hands to my ears to hear at her chosen level. It finally dawned on me that maybe it isn't just the Alzheimer's disease. Maybe I have a hearing problem. At my annual checkup last month, I asked my internist to refer me for an audiogram. It showed severe hearing loss on the left in the higher frequencies and moderate loss in the lower frequencies. The right ear wasn't quite as bad with severe hearing loss only in the higher frequencies and normal hearing in the lower and midrange frequencies.

Almost everyone experiences hearing loss with age, particularly in the high frequencies. This affects our ability to hear and understand speech, especially the speech of females. By age 80, most people have significant hearing impairment. I'm just about ten years ahead of that usual, auditory decline, especially in the left ear. The audiologist recommended that I get fitted for hearing aids. I am put off a bit by the anticipated hassle of using these devices, but I plan to look into it more soon.

An increasing number of studies have shown that hearing loss may be a modifiable risk factor for all-cause dementia. There is agreement that people with significant hearing loss are more likely to develop dementia than those with normal hearing [1], but there is uncertainty about whether treatment of hearing loss would reduce the risk of developing dementia. Several recent studies appear to show that the use of hearing aids can indeed reduce the risk of dementia in hearing-impaired subjects. In a 2021 study published in *Alzheimer's & Dementia* [2], hearing-impaired subjects with MCI who wore hearing aids were 27% less likely to progress to dementia compared to those who did not wear hearing aids. A much larger meta-analysis of eight studies including 126,903 subjects with hearing loss showed a significant 19% lower chance of developing dementia in those who used hearing aids compared to those that didn't [3].

I was slow to come around, but I am now convinced that there is a very good chance that hearing aids will not only improve my hearing and my ability to understand speech, but perhaps also slow the progression of my Alzheimer's disease.

References

1   Huang AR, Jiang K, Lin FR, Deal JA, Reed NS. Hearing loss and dementia prevalence in older adults in the US. *JAMA* 2023; 329: 171–173. https://doi.org/10.1001/jama.2022.20954.

2   Bucholc M, McClean PL, Bauermeister S, *et al.* Association of the use of hearing aids with the conversion from mild cognitive impairment to dementia and progression of dementia: A longitudinal retrospective study. *Alzheimers Dement* 2021; 7: e12122. https://doi.org/10.1002/trc2.12122 (open access).
3   Yeo BSY, Song HJJMD, Toh EMS, *et al.* Association of hearing aids and cochlear implants with cognitive decline and dementia: A systematic review and meta-analysis. *JAMA Neurol* 2023; 80: 134–141. https://doi.org/10.1001/jamaneurol.2022.4427.

26 TO SLEEP, PERCHANCE TO DREAM

A number of studies have previously noted that people with dementia tend to sleep less than those without dementia. The question has been what is cause and what is effect? Does getting less sleep promote the onset of dementia or does dementia disrupt sleep? The answer appears to be that both are true.

Sleep disorders are an almost universal problem with moderate and advanced dementia, especially for those with Alzheimer's disease. Sometimes these issues can occur even before there is cognitive impairment. About a year before I was diagnosed with MCI due to Alzheimer's disease, Lois noticed that I would jerk my legs during sleep, making a scratching sound on the sheets. She even tried to hold my leg down, but it continued to jerk. These spells occurred about every 20 seconds and were most likely due to periodic limb movement disorder (PLMD), a type of sleep myoclonus (rhythmic muscle jerks). PLMD can be associated with other sleep disorders such as restless leg syndrome. Lois did a Google search and found that PLMD can also be an early sign of cognitive impairment [1], so she chose not to tell me about my jerking legs until later because she knew I was worried about incipient Alzheimer's.

People living with Alzheimer's disease often have trouble falling asleep and staying asleep, especially in the later stages. The sleep–wake cycle may be reversed. People with advanced Alzheimer's lie awake an average of 40% of the time in bed at night and then spend a significant part of the day asleep. When awake at night, they may wander or yell out, disrupting the sleep of caregivers as well. Sleep problems can also be exacerbated by depression, restless leg syndrome, and sleep apnea, all of which are common in Alzheimer's and other dementias.

Some medications can also disrupt sleep. Cholinesterase inhibitors such as donepezil (Aricept) are taken by many people with Alzheimer's disease, but if taken at bedtime they often cause vivid nightmares. I experienced this myself within a few weeks of starting the medication and discovered that it is a well-recognized side effect. When I switched to taking it in the morning, I stopped having nightmares. A few days ago, I got my medications mixed up and took the donepezil at bedtime instead of in the morning, and sure enough, I was chased throughout the night by gunmen trying to kill me.

So, Alzheimer's and medications can disrupt sleep, but does lack of sleep affect the risk of getting Alzheimer's? This has been surprisingly difficult to determine. A report in *Nature Communications* provides the most compelling answer yet. The Whitehall II study was started in the 1980s in the UK as a long-term investigation of various risk factors for a variety of diseases. Nearly 8,000 subjects in this study were recruited when they were about 50 years of age and asked about nightly sleep duration at age 50, 60, and 70. At age 70, 6,875 of these subjects were still alive and free of dementia. Over the next seven years, 426 of these subjects developed dementia. Those who slept six or fewer hours each night at age 50 and 60 were about 30% more likely to develop dementia by the time they were 77 than those who reported sleeping seven or more hours per night. The authors concluded "that short sleep duration in midlife is associated with the higher risk of dementia later in life, independently of sociodemographic, behavioral, cardiometabolic, and mental health factors"[2].

Why might getting adequate sleep be important in reducing the risk of dementia, especially Alzheimer's?

As I describe in *A Tattoo on my Brain*, a number of studies in animals and humans have suggested that beta-amyloid and other toxins are removed from the brain during sleep by a fluid similar to cerebrospinal fluid (CSF) [3]. The flow of this cleansing fluid through the spaces surrounding small blood vessels in the brain, the so-called glymphatic circulation, is most active during non-REM, slow-wave sleep and is driven by a combination of brain electrical activity and arterial pulsations [4].

Getting adequate sleep during midlife is really important for reducing the risk of dementia including Alzheimer's disease. Remember, the pathological changes of Alzheimer's, especially the amyloid plaques, can start forming 20 years before there is any cognitive impairment. This is the time, when we are in our 50s and maybe even our 40s, when it is especially important to get at least seven hours of sleep every night.

What about getting too much sleep? An interesting paper in *JAMA Neurology* suggests that the relationship between sleep and cognitive impairment may be more complicated than we realized [5]. Over 4,000 subjects without clinical dementia aged 65–85 years were screened with amyloid PET scans and cognitive tests. Those reporting sleeping less than seven hours per night did significantly worse on memory tests than those getting eight hours. They also had more amyloid in their brains. Surprisingly (at least to me), those getting excessive sleep, more than nine hours nightly, also had more amyloid in their brains, and they did worse on tests of executive function such as making plans. The under- and over-sleepers both had signs of poor health such as an increased body mass index. For me, this makes the sleep question more complicated. Are they sleeping less or more because of other health issues, issues that might independently increase the risk for amyloid deposition and Alzheimer's disease, or is the eight-hour target really ideal for maximizing brain health? More studies will be needed to sort this out, but in the meantime, as my mother tried to convince me, use moderation in all things.

References

1 Leng Y, Blackwell T, Stone KL, *et al*. Periodic limb movements in sleep are associated with greater cognitive decline in older men without dementia. *Sleep* 2016; 39: 1807–1810. https://doi.org/10.5665/sleep.6158. PMID: 27568800; PMCID: PMC5020362 (open access).

2 Sabia S, Fayosse A, Dumurgier J, *et al*. Association of sleep duration in middle and old age with incidence of dementia. *Nat Commun* 2021; 12: 2289. https://doi.org/10.1038/s41467-021-22354-2 (open access).

3 Gibbs DM, Barker TH. *A Tattoo on my Brain: A Neurologist's Personal Battle against Alzheimer's Disease* (second edition). Cambridge: Cambridge University Press, 2023, pp. 111–112.

4 Fultz NE, Bonmassar G, Setsompop K, *et al*. Coupled electrophysiological, hemodynamic, and cerebrospinal fluid oscillations in human sleep. *Science* 2019; 366: 628–631. https://doi.org/10.1126/science.aax5440.

5 Winer JR, Deters KD, Kennedy G, *et al*. Association of short and long sleep duration with amyloid-β burden and cognition in aging. *JAMA Neurol* 2021; 78: 1187–1196. https://doi.org/10.1001/jamaneurol.2021.2876.

27 THE AMYLOID HYPOTHESIS IS NOT DEAD, BUT IT MAY BE GASPING FOR BREATH

The amyloid hypothesis has been the dominant theory for the cause of Alzheimer's disease for over 20 years. In brief, the theory holds that Alzheimer's disease is caused by the accumulation of beta-amyloid that damages nerve cells in the brain. Beta-amyloid is cleaved from the large amyloid precursor protein (APP) into two main peptides that are released outside the cell, beta-amyloid 40 and beta-amyloid 42, containing respectively 40 and 42 amino acids. According to the amyloid hypothesis, in normal people, these peptides are rapidly removed, but in people with Alzheimer's disease the metabolic ability to degrade them is decreased, the peptides accumulate, form fibrils, and ultimately solid amyloid plaques that in turn damage neurons and trigger the formation of abnormal tau pathology causing neuronal death. There certainly is no doubt that amyloid plaques and tau-containing neurofibrillary tangles exist in Alzheimer's disease. The question is are they causative or are they simply the debris left over as the disease progresses for other reasons? Soluble beta-amyloid is neurotoxic in mouse models of Alzheimer's, but there is increasing unease that things are not as simple as the amyloid hypothesis would suggest [1]. From 1995 through 2021, many drug trials costing an estimated total of $42.5 billion failed to show a significant reversal or even slowing of disease progression in Alzheimer's patients [2]. Some of these drugs have been very effective in removing amyloid plaques, but as of 2022, only one, lecanemab, has demonstrated a modest but statistically significant slowing of cognitive deterioration [3]. Lecanemab might be that gasp of air that will save the amyloid hypothesis. I will go into it in more detail in the following chapter. Another drug, aducanumab, showed modest slowing of cognitive decline in only one of two parallel trials reported in 2021 [4]. In a very controversial ruling, the FDA approved the release of aducanumab for treating Alzheimer's disease despite the objections of many Alzheimer's experts.

The failure of most of these anti-amyloid drugs to date has been blamed by some on giving them too late. The idea is that once cognitive impairment has started, there has already been death of neurons, and they cannot be replaced. This has led to several trials of anti-amyloid drugs in subjects with presymptomatic Alzheimer's disease. These research subjects have positive biomarkers for Alzheimer's such as amyloid and/or tau PET scans or blood tests, but they do not yet have any cognitive impairment. Two of these presymptomatic anti-amyloid drug trials have already failed, including the trial of crenezumab in the Colombian kindred with the autosomal dominant *prescnilin-1* mutation [5], and the trial of solanezumab that did not slow the progression of cognitive decline due to Alzheimer's disease pathology when initiated in individuals with PET scan evidence of amyloid plaques but no clinical symptoms of the disease [6]. The results of the other studies will start to appear over the next few years. Lecanemab and donenumab may have the best chance for success in these presymptomatic trials as they are both extremely effective at removing amyloid plaques from the brain.

The frustration at failing to find effective anti-amyloid medications for Alzheimer's received a bombshell recently with the publication in *Science* [7] of a six-month investigative study that alleges falsified data in a 2006 study published in *Nature* [8] that was an important lynchpin for the amyloid hypothesis. The authors of that *Nature* paper claimed to have isolated a 56-kilodalton soluble beta-amyloid assembly from the brains of cognitively impaired, transgenic mice carrying human DNA coding for human *APP*. They called this isolate Aβ*56. When they injected purified Aβ*56 into the brains of young, healthy rats, the rats became cognitively impaired. The authors proposed that "... Aβ*56 impairs memory independently of plaques or neuronal loss, and may contribute to cognitive deficits associated with Alzheimer's disease." This appeared to be very strong evidence that a soluble beta-amyloid fragment could by itself cause the neuronal damage found in Alzheimer's disease. According to experts in the field, working with amyloid fragments is technically difficult as they can be very unstable, so it was not particularly alarming that this work could not be replicated by others. The investigation conducted for *Science* found evidence of data falsification in the *Nature* paper, calling into question the validity of other papers based on these results.

I have not totally given up on the amyloid hypothesis. There is still evidence that some forms of beta-amyloid can be neurotoxic, but even this basic tenet of the amyloid hypothesis has become controversial. Dr. Alberto Espay and his collaborators have argued that Alzheimer's disease may not be caused by increased levels of toxic beta-amyloid but rather by the *reduction* of a soluble, *protective* form of beta-amyloid:

> The spread of brain amyloidosis can be fully explained by mechanisms of spontaneous or catalyzed polymerization and phase transformation instead of active replication .... Early neuronal toxicity in Alzheimer's disease may therefore be mediated to a greater extent

by a reduction in the pool of soluble, normal-functioning protein than its accumulation in the polymerized state [9].

I suspect that the causes of neuronal loss and dementia in Alzheimer's will turn out to be more complicated than we previously thought. According to Dr. Grace Stutzmann's comment after an *Alzforum* article about the Aβ*56 fiasco (one of 31 comments): "We also see the rise of alternative mechanisms independent of amyloid pathology, including neuroinflammatory cascades, synaptic pathophysiology, calcium mishandling, and mitochondrial dysfunction — none of which are mutually exclusive" [10]. Clearly, we have much more to learn before we fully understand the neurobiology of Alzheimer's disease.

References

1   Kametani F, Hasegawa M. Reconsideration of amyloid hypothesis and tau hypothesis in Alzheimer's disease. *Front Neurosci* 2018; 12: 25. https://doi.org/10.3389/fnins.2018.00025. PMID: 29440986; PMCID: PMC5797629 (open access).

2   Cummings JL, Goldman DP, Simmons-Stern NR, Ponton E. The costs of developing treatments for Alzheimer's disease: A retrospective exploration. *Alzheimers Dement* 2021; 18: 469–477. https://doi.org/10.1002/alz.12450 (open access).

3   Van Dyck CH, Swanson CJ, Aisen P, *et al.* Lecanemab in early Alzheimer's disease. *N Engl J Med* 2023; 388: 9–21. https://doi.org/10.1056/NEJMoa2212948

4   Knopman DS, Jones DT, Greicius MD. Failure to demonstrate efficacy of aducanumab: An analysis of the EMERGE and ENGAGE trials as reported by Biogen, December 2019. *Alzheimers Dement* 2021; 17: 696–701. https://doi.org/10.1002/alz.12213 (open access).

5   Rogers MB. API Colombian trial of crenezumab missed primary endpoints. *Alzforum*. June 18, 2022. www .alzforum.org/news/research-news/api-colombian-trial-crenezumab-missed-primary-endpoints (open access)

6   Eli Lilly and Company Press Release. Update on A4 study of solanezumab for preclinical Alzheimer's disease. March 8, 2023. https://a4study.org/study-results/ (open access).

7   Piller C. Blots on a field? *Science* 2022; 377: 358–363. www.science.org/content/article/potential-fabrication-research-images-threatens-key-theory-alzheimers-disease (open access).

8   Lesné S, Koh M, Kotilinek L, *et al.* A specific amyloid-β protein assembly in the brain impairs memory. *Nature* 2006; 440: 352–357. https://doi.org/10.1038/nature04533.

9   Espay AJ, Sturchio A, Schneider LS, Ezzat K. Soluble amyloid-β consumption in Alzheimer's disease. *J Alzheimers Dis* 2021; 82(4): 1403–1415. https://doi.org/10.3233/JAD-210415; PMID: 34151810.

10   Rogers MB. Sylvain Lesné, who found Aβ*56, accused of image manipulation. *Alzforum*. July 22, 2022; see comment by Dr. Grace Stutzmann. www.alzforum.org/news/community-news/sylvain-lesne-who-found-av56-accused-image-manipulation (open access).

28 COULD LECANEMAB OFFER A RAY OF HOPE?

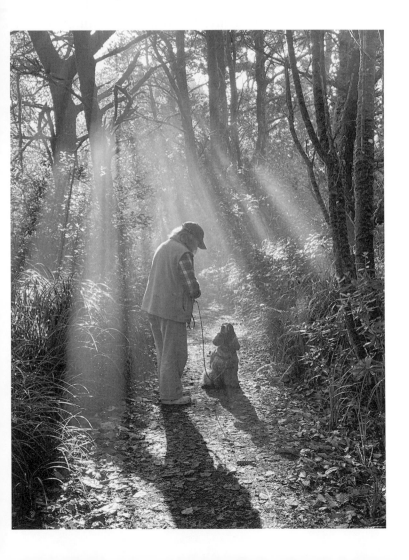

Many drugs designed to remove beta-amyloid from the brains of people with Alzheimer's disease have been designed and tested over the last 20–30 years. Most of these have been very effective in animal models of Alzheimer's, but results in humans have been frustratingly negative in reversing or even slowing cognitive decline. Some of the drugs such as donanemab are very good at removing beta-amyloid plaques from the brain, but none of these have significantly slowed cognitive decline. Aducanumab came tantalizing close with mild slowing of cognitive impairment in one of two identical phase 3 trials, but there was no benefit in the other trial. Although aducanumab was approved by the FDA, its use outside of further clinical trials remains controversial.

In January 2023, researchers from Eisai and its partner Biogen published positive results in a phase 3 trial of the anti-amyloid monoclonal antibody lecanemab. All research subjects had either mild cognitive impairment or early dementia due to Alzheimer's disease. The primary endpoint was the Clinical Dementia Rating – Sum of Boxes (CDR-SB). This is a numeric scale used to quantify the severity of symptoms of dementia. It is based on interviews of people living with dementia and their caregivers by qualified professionals who assess cognitive and functional performance in six areas: memory, orientation, judgment and problem solving, community affairs, home and hobbies, and personal care. The total score of the six areas is the score of the CDR-SB. After 18 months, those receiving lecanemab had 27% less decline of the CDR-SB compared to those receiving a placebo. This was highly significant statistically ($p = 0.00005$). Brain swelling (ARIA-E) occurred in 12.3% of subjects, about one third the occurrence rate seen in the aducanumab phase 3 trials [1]. However, participants with two copies of the *APOE-4* allele were approximately six times more likely to experience symptomatic ARIA with brain swelling and more than three times more likely to experience ARIA with brain bleeding than *APOE-4* noncarriers [2].

Why should lecanemab be more effective than any of the other anti-amyloid monoclonal antibodies (MAB) tested so far? Early anti-amyloid MABs such as crenezumab targeted soluble beta-amyloid whereas more recent anti-amyloid MABs such as aducanumab, gantenerumab, and donanemab bind most firmly to aggregated amyloid in plaques. Lecanemab uniquely binds to an intermediate form called protofibril amyloid that is found in astrocytes, important support cells in the brain. Interestingly, the development of lecanemab was based on the discovery of the rare "Arctic" mutation in the gene for *APP*. This mutation causes a disease clinically identical to Alzheimer's except that it is associated with high levels of amyloid protofibrils and the relative absence of amyloid plaques [3]. This suggested that the amyloid protofibrils might be the real culprits in Alzheimer's, not the amyloid plaques.

Is lecanemab a breakthrough? It may well be. It is the first drug so far to show unambiguous slowing of cognitive impairment in early Alzheimer's disease. Some have said that the beneficial effect may be too small to be noticed by the patient and family, and it may be less effective and more dangerous to use in *APOE-4* carriers. It is not a cure for Alzheimer's. But it is an exciting first step, and the amyloid hypothesis seems to have been thrown a timely lifeline just as drowning had appeared imminent.

As this book goes to print, Eli Lilly and Co. just announced in a press release encouraging results of a phase 3 clinical trial of their anti-amyloid MAB donanemab. Donanemab is unique among anti-amyloid MABs as it specifically targets N-terminally truncated pyroglutamate-modified beta-amyloid (AβpE), a form of beta-amyloid apparently found only in amyloid plaques. The primary endpoint (integrated Alzheimer's Disease Rating Scale, or iADRS) showed 35% slowing of decline compared to placebo and a secondary endpoint (Clinical Dementia Rating-Sum of Boxes, or CDR-SB) showed 36% slowing of decline over 18 months. In addition, nearly half (47%) of the participants on donanemab, compared to 29% on a placebo, showed no clinical progression at one year as defined by an absence of decline in the CDR-SB score. These results suggest that donanemab may be more effective at slowing cognitive decline in Alzheimer's disease than other anti-amyloid MABs previously trialed. However, the report that three participants died during or following severe ARIA events is of concern. More information is expected at the July 2023 Alzheimer's Association International Conference in Amsterdam and in peer reviewed publications.

References

1   van Dyck CH, Swanson CJ, Aisen P, *et al*. Lecanemab in early Alzheimer's disease. *N Engl J Med* 2023; 388: 9–21. https://doi.org/10.1056/NEJMoa2212948.

2   Thambisetty M, Howard R. Lecanemab and APOE genotyping in clinical practice — navigating uncharted terrain. *JAMA Neurol* 2023; published online March 13. https://doi.org/10.1001/jamaneurol.2023.0207.

3   Nilsberth C, Westlind-Danielsson A, Eckman C, *et al*. The 'Arctic' APP mutation (E693G) causes Alzheimer's disease by enhanced Aβ protofibril formation. *Nature Neurosci* 2001; 4: 887–893. https://doi.org/10.1038/nn0901-887.

29 A FATAL CASE OF MULTIPLE BRAIN HEMORRHAGES ASSOCIATED WITH LECANEMAB

On January 6, 2023, the FDA granted accelerated approval of the anti-amyloid monoclonal antibody lecanemab, now going by the trade name Leqembi. I have mixed feelings about this. Lecanemab is the only disease-modifying drug so far to show statistically significant slowing of cognitive impairment in subjects with mild Alzheimer's disease, and it is very effective in removing beta-amyloid from the brain. This is exciting. On the other hand, while the slowing of cognitive impairment was statistically significant, it was modest (27%) and might not be recognizable by patients or their families. It is quite possible that this drug may be more effective if started earlier, and in fact a trial in subjects with pre-symptomatic Alzheimer's, the AHEAD Trial, is already underway [1]. I am keeping my fingers crossed that the AHEAD Trial will ultimately show that lecanemab can meaningfully slow or even prevent the onset of Alzheimer's symptoms in these subjects who already have evidence of Alzheimer's pathology in their brains.

However, there is a darker side to anti-amyloid MABs including lecanemab. ARIA, an acronym for amyloid-related imaging abnormalities, have occurred in all trials of anti-amyloid MABs. They occur in two forms, swelling (edema) of the brain (ARIA-E) and microhemorrhages

(ARIA-H). Most of the time they are harmless and without symptoms, and they usually resolve within a month or two after stopping the drug. Rarely, they can be severe. As described in a case study, I was one of the subjects in the aducanumab trial who had severe ARIA of both types, swelling and bleeding. I required ICU care for two days, but I eventually fully recovered over the next few months [2].

So far, three research subjects have died during the lecanemab clinical trial. Biogen has stated that the deaths were not caused by receiving lecanemab, but a case study of one of these deaths was published recently as a letter in the *New England Journal of Medicine* and suggests otherwise [3]. The patient was a 65-year-old woman with mild Alzheimer's disease who had received three doses of lecanemab as part of the open label extension phase of the trial. It is not publicly known if she received active lecanemab or placebo during the preceding double-blind portion of the trial. She was seen in an emergency room 30 minutes after the sudden onset of inability to speak (expressive aphasia) and a left gaze preference (eyes forcibly tuned to the left). A CT scan showed evidence of an acute, ischemic stroke in the left temporal-parietal region of her brain and blockage of a distal branch of the left middle cerebral artery, the principal source of blood flow to much of the frontal and parietal lobes. There were no hemorrhages visible at the time of the CT scan. She received the clot-buster tissue plasminogen activator (t-PA) for treatment of her acute, ischemic stroke. During the t-PA infusion, her condition worsened. An MRI showed multiple, large areas of new bleeding on both sides of her brain. She subsequently died, and at autopsy, she had extensive hemorrhages with swelling throughout her brain.

She also had beta-amyloid deposition in the walls of the small blood vessels of her brain as well as the typical amyloid plaques and neurofibrillary tangles of Alzheimer's disease. This amyloid within the walls of the brain blood vessels is called cerebral amyloid angiopathy (CAA), and is one of the major causes of brain hemorrhages in the elderly.

Based on autopsy evidence, CAA is found in 48% of subjects with Alzheimer's pathology in the brain. Unfortunately, there are limited ways to assess CAA during life. An indirect measure is based on the presence of microhemorrhages seen on blood-sensitive MRI scans, but this is much less sensitive as these are found in only 22% of people with Alzheimer's disease [4]. This suggests that our only test for CAA in the living has a sensitivity of less than 50%. The patient who died after receiving lecanemab along with the clot-buster t-PA had autopsy proven CAA, but she had no microhemorrhages at the beginning of the lecanemab study. I had no sign of microhemorrhages before my ARIA episode, but I almost certainly have CAA.

In my opinion, patients who have known CAA should not receive anti-amyloid MABs such as lecanemab or aducanumab, and they should be given clot-busting drugs such as t-PA only with great caution. We really need more sensitive biomarkers for CAA. The presence of microhemorrhages on MRI is not good enough.

References

1   AHEAD Study. Lecanemab for people with increased risk of Alzheimer's disease. www.alzheimers.gov/clinical-trials/ahead-study-ban2401-people-increased-risk-alzheimers-disease (accessed 2/12/2023).

2   VandeVrede L, Gibbs DM, Koestler M, *et al*. Symptomatic amyloid-related imaging abnormalities in an APOE ε4/ε4 patient treated with aducanumab. *Alzheimers Dement* 2020; 12: e12101. https://doi.org/10.1002/dad2.12101 (open access).

3   Reish NJ, Jamshidi P, Stamm B, *et al*. Multiple cerebral hemorrhages in a patient receiving lecanemab and

treated with t-PA for stroke. *N Engl J Med* 2023; 388: 478. https://doi.org/10.1056/NEJMc2215148.

4   Jäkel L, Anna M, De Kort AM, Schreuder FHBM, *et al.* Prevalence of cerebral amyloid angiopathy: A systematic review and meta-analysis. *Alzheimers Dement* 2022, 18: 10–28. https://doi.org/10.1002/alz.12366 (open access).

30 CEREBRAL AMYLOID ANGIOPATHY (CAA)

Should It Be a Contraindication for Drugs Like Lecanemab?

Early in my career as a neurologist, probably about 1990, I was asked to consult on a 62-year-old, previously healthy woman who had had a large brain hemorrhage. She had no apparent risk factors such as high blood pressure, head trauma, aneurysms, tumors, or anticoagulants such as warfarin, and she had no cognitive impairment suggestive of dementia. She had a good recovery from the brain hemorrhage and was able to return to her job as an office manager. Two years later she had a second bleeding episode in a different lobe of her brain. This time she had cognitive problems that did not improve. An angiogram of her cerebral arteries and veins showed no abnormalities. A spinal tap showed elevated protein and white blood cells in her spinal fluid suggesting the possibility of inflammation in her brain, so I recommended treatment with steroids thinking she might have primary CNS vasculitis, an inflammatory disease of the cerebral blood vessels. The steroids didn't help, and she became progressively impaired and died a year later. The autopsy revealed that she had cerebral amyloid angiopathy (CAA), and she also had many amyloid plaques and tau-containing neurofibrillary tangles throughout her brain consistent with Alzheimer's disease.

CAA is vascular disease of the brain in which beta-amyloid is deposited in the walls of small arteries and capillaries. The amyloid replaces smooth muscle cells causing vessel wall thickening and stiffness. This can result in leaks and reduced blood flow in these small blood vessels. Tiny hemorrhages and small strokes are seen surrounding the affected blood vessels. In the elderly, CAA is a major cause of serious bleeding in the various lobes of the brain. Genetically, it can occur sporadically or in families. There is often but not always an overlap with Alzheimer's disease. The beta-amyloid in vessel walls in CAA is usually the shorter peptide fragment, Aβ40 (40 amino acids in length), compared to that in the amyloid plaques of Alzheimer's disease, Aβ42. Pathological evidence of CAA is found in over half of brains that have Alzheimer's amyloid plaques and neurofibrillary tangles [1].

Although the first symptom of CAA can be a catastrophic brain hemorrhage in an elderly patient, personality changes, particularly apathy, may occur much earlier. As in Alzheimer's disease, apathy in CAA appears to be caused by damage to neural circuits in the prefrontal cortex [2]. In the absence of major bleeding or a biopsy, CAA is surprisingly difficult to detect during life. Currently, the best noninvasive test is an MRI protocol called susceptibility weighted imaging (SWI). This is an MRI technique that is particularly sensitive to blood and other iron-containing compounds that distort the local magnetic field. Although the SWI-MRI is not completely specific for blood, the distribution of these black dots around blood vessels correlates very well with the presence at autopsy of microhemorrhages associated with CAA. Although SWI-MRI is the best test for CAA at present, it can only detect CAA if there has been leakage of blood from these damaged blood vessels. The location and number of so-called white matter hyperintensities as seen on FLAIR MRI images may also support the diagnosis [3]. The sensitivity of these MRI techniques for detecting CAA is probably about half that of examining the brain at autopsy. We really can't yet detect the early stages of CAA during life.

Although there is no treatment for CAA, people who have it are at increased risk for major bleeding in the brain. In patients with a known history or even a suspicion of CAA, I believe that anti-amyloid monoclonal antibodies such as lecanemab should not be given. People who have had ARIA-H (amyloid-related imaging abnormalities with microhemorrhages) during treatment with an anti-amyloid

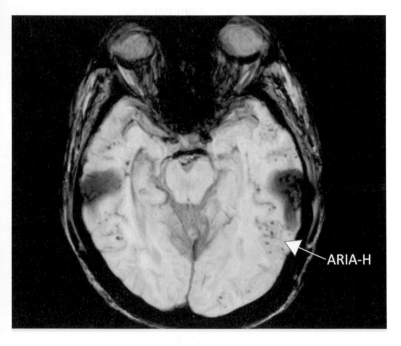

This is a susceptibility weighted MRI during my 2017 ARIA episode showing multiple, bilateral microhemorrhages in my temporal lobes. The microhemorrhages (ARIA-H) appear as black dots, mostly clustered around blood vessels. They are closely related if not identical to microhemorrhages associated with cerebral amyloid angiopathy (CAA).

monoclonal antibody may have CAA, and they should be closely monitored by MRI if the drug is continued. Caution should also be used in the use of blood-thinning drugs such as warfarin or the clot-busting medication tissue plasminogen activator (t-PA) as these may increase the chance of a potentially fatal hemorrhage in those with CAA [4,5].

References

1 Viswanathan A, Greenberg SM. Cerebral amyloid angiopathy in the elderly. *Ann Neurol* 2011; 70: 871–880. https://doi.org/10.1002/ana.22516 (open access).

2 Chokesuwattanaskul A, Zotin MCZ, Schoemaker D, *et al*. Apathy in patients with cerebral amyloid angiopathy: A multimodal neuroimaging study. *Neurology* 2023 (published online ahead of print on March 20, 2023). https://doi.org/10.1212/WNL.0000000000207200.

3 Kozberg MG, Perosa V, Gurol ME, van Veluw SJ. A practical approach to the management of cerebral amyloid angiopathy. *Int J Stroke* 2021; 16: 356–369. https://doi.org/10.1177/1747493020974464 (open access).

4 Rosand J, Hylek EM, O'Donnell HC, Greenberg SM. Warfarin-associated hemorrhage and cerebral amyloid angiopathy: A genetic and pathologic study. *Neurology* 2000; 55: 947–951. https://doi.org/10.1212/wnl.55.7.947. PMID: 11061249.

5 Reish NJ, Jamshidi P, Stamm B, *et al*. Multiple cerebral hemorrhages in a patient receiving lecanemab and treated with t-PA for stroke. *N Engl J Med* 2023; 388: 478. https://doi.org/10.1056/NEJMc2215148.

31 HITTING THE SWEET SPOT IN THE SPECTRUM OF ALZHEIMER'S DISEASE FOR FUTURE TRIALS OF ANTI-AMYLOID MEDICATIONS

Evidence of beta-amyloid plaques can be found in the brains of people up to 20 years prior to the onset of cognitive impairment due to Alzheimer's disease and yet, some people with beta-amyloid plaques will never develop Alzheimer's. Abnormal tau protein starts to appear in neurofibrillary tangles in the brain later but still at least several years before the onset of cognitive impairment. Information from amyloid and tau PET scans as well as new blood tests for beta-amyloid and tau have confirmed this timeline.

As we have seen, attempts to treat Alzheimer's disease by removing beta-amyloid have almost all failed. Some of these medications have been very effective at removing beta-amyloid, but all but one, lecanemab, have failed to significantly slow the progression of cognitive impairment in subjects with MCI or mild Alzheimer's dementia. Several recent trials are studying the effects of these drugs earlier in the disease, before there has been any cognitive impairment. All subjects in these trials must have biomarker evidence of brain amyloid as well as normal cognition. These trials require a positive amyloid PET scan and/or one of the new sensitive and specific blood tests for beta-amyloid to qualify participants for the study. Although I am very excited about these "preventative" trials and I really hope they succeed, there is an intrinsic problem. If the asymptomatic amyloid-positive phase of Alzheimer's can last up to 20 years, how will we know if removing the amyloid will prevent or slow Alzheimer's disease? It is impractical to wait 20 years to find out. Ideally, we should be studying subjects who are amyloid-positive, don't yet have tau in their brains, but will become tau-positive within a few years.

A recent paper in *Neurology* shows how it might be possible to identify research subjects who are in this narrow window, those who currently have amyloid but no tau, but who have characteristics suggesting that they will become tau-positive and cognitively impaired within five years [1]. These investigators at the Mayo Clinic collected data from the Alzheimer's Disease Neuroimaging Initiative, a large, international database containing amyloid and tau PET scans and MRIs obtained from hundreds of subjects representing all stages of the Alzheimer's spectrum. While all subjects had detectable brain amyloid but no tau at the outset, those with higher levels of amyloid, atrophy of the hippocampus seen on MRI, *APOE-4* positivity, and less preserved cognition were significantly more likely to have a positive tau PET scan and/or dementia in five years. Restricting participants in trials of anti-amyloid medications to those with a higher amyloid burden, smaller hippocampi, and *APOE-4* positivity could be important for proof of concept: Can anti-amyloid medications slow or even stop the progression of pre-symptomatic Alzheimer's disease? If such a trial were to yield negative results, it would probably be the final nail in the coffin for anti-amyloid therapies. But, if these trials of anti-amyloid medications restricted to those on the verge of converting to tau-positivity and cognitive impairment were positive, it will be a great leap forward, and further studies with broader inclusion criteria could begin.

References

1   Josephs KA, Weigand SD, Whitwell JL. Characterizing amyloid-positive individuals with normal tau PET levels after 5 years: An ADNI study. *Neurology* 2022; 98: e2282–e2292. https://doi.org/10.1212/WNL.0000000000 200287; Epub 2022 Mar 21. PMID: 35314506; PMCID: PMC9162162 (open access).

32 DISAPPOINTING RESULTS OF TWO HUMAN TRIALS OF MONOCLONAL ANTIBODIES IN PARKINSON'S DISEASE

Like Alzheimer's disease, Parkinson's disease is a progressive, neurodegenerative disorder that involves deposits of an abnormal protein in the brain. In Alzheimer's disease, these abnormal proteins are extracellular beta-amyloid and intraneuronal, hyperphosphorylated tau. In Parkinson's disease, the neuropathological findings are protein deposits of aggregated alpha-synuclein found primarily within neurons in a part of the brainstem called the substantia nigra but in other locations as well. These clumps of alpha-synuclein are called Lewy bodies.

Although Parkinson's disease can certainly cause dementia in the late stages, early symptoms usually involve trouble with movement. For many, the first problem is an intermittent tremor while at rest, usually on one side. The tremor goes away when the arm is used and may get worse while walking. Handwriting may get very tiny (micrographia). Balance is usually affected, and an unsteady, shuffling gait may be an early sign of the disease. Interestingly, as in Alzheimer's disease, many people with Parkinson's disease experience a decreased sense of smell years before any other symptoms occur, and Lewy bodies can be found in the olfactory bulb very early in the disease. For those wanting more details about the putative role of alpha-synuclein and Lewy bodies in Parkinson's disease, I recommend this excellent and comprehensive, open-access review paper [1].

In animal models of both Alzheimer's disease and Parkinson's disease, therapies directed at removing these abnormal protein deposits have shown success in halting progression of the clinical manifestations of disease. However, at least in Alzheimer's disease, human trials conducted for medications designed to remove beta-amyloid or tau from the brain have almost all failed to show meaningful slowing of cognitive decline despite being effective at removing the targeted protein. The only convincing exception so far is the anti-amyloid monoclonal antibody, lecanemab, that demonstrated a mild but statistically significant slowing of cognitive impairment in subjects with MCI or mild Alzheimer's dementia [2]. All anti-amyloid monoclonal antibodies thus far have targeted either the soluble form or the aggregated (solid) form of amyloid. Lecanemab uniquely targets an intermediate, protofibril form of amyloid and this may be the key to its possible success.

In the August 4, 2022 issue of the *New England Journal of Medicine*, we now have reports of two phase 2 human trials of monoclonal antibodies directed at alpha-synuclein in subjects with early-stage Parkinson's disease, prasinezumab [3] and cinpanemab [4]. The subjects were treated for at least 52 weeks with either active drug or placebo. Mild side effects were common in both studies, mostly at the time of the monthly infusions, but no serious side effects were encountered. Disappointingly, no significant benefits were seen with either drug for primary and secondary endpoints compared to subjects receiving a placebo.

What is the take home message here? I think nearly everyone in the field is frustrated. Multiple animal studies have shown beneficial effects of targeting these abnormal proteins in the brain, beta-amyloid and tau in Alzheimer's disease and now, alpha-synuclein in Parkinson's disease. But, with one exception, lecanemab in early-stage Alzheimer's disease, none of the monoclonal antibodies or other drugs targeting these proteins have shown any significant, clinical benefit in humans. Several of the anti-amyloid monoclonal antibodies including the FDA-approved aducanumab are very effective in removing amyloid plaques from the brain, but so far, almost all of them have failed to show efficacy in slowing cognitive decline. Some researchers feel that we have been barking up the wrong tree and that we need to change course [5]. Others are proposing that these drugs may still be helpful if started earlier in the disease, perhaps even before any symptoms have occurred. Hopefully, we will learn from these failures and discover new paths toward successful treatments of Alzheimer's, Parkinson's, and the other neurodegenerative disorders, but there is still a lot of work to do.

References

1   Fields CR, Bengoa-Vergniory N, Wade-Martins R. Targeting alpha-synuclein as a therapy for Parkinson's disease. *Front Mol Neurosci* 2019; 12: 299. https://doi.org/10.3389/fnmol.2019.00299 (open access).

2   van Dyck CH, Swanson CJ, Aisen P, *et al*. Lecanemab in early Alzheimer's disease. *N Engl J Med* 2023; 388: 9–21. https://doi.org/10.1056/NEJMoa2212948.

3   Pagano G, Taylor KI, Anzures-Cabrera J, *et al*. Trial of prasinezumab in early-stage Parkinson's disease. *N Engl*

J Med 2022; 387: 421–432. https://doi.org/10.1056/
NEJMoa2202867.

4   Lang AE, Siderowf AD, Macklin EA, *et al.* Trial of cinpanemab in early Parkinson's disease. *N Engl J Med* 2022;
387: 408–420. https://doi.org/10.1056/NEJMoa2203395.

5   Espay AJ, Okun MS. Abandoning the proteinopathy
paradigm in Parkinson's disease. *JAMA Neurol* 2023; 80:
123–124. https://doi.org/10.1001/jamaneurol.2022.4193.

33 REPURPOSING OLD DRUGS FOR ALZHEIMER'S TREATMENT

We've talked a lot about clinical trials of several so-called disease-modifying drugs for Alzheimer's disease. These are medications designed to slow and perhaps even stop the progression of the disease. Most of them so far have been drugs that remove beta-amyloid from the brain or block its production. Almost all of the clinical trials of these anti-amyloid drugs have been disappointing, although recently lecanemab received accelerated approval by the FDA based on effectiveness of removing amyloid plaques from the brain and a 27% slowing of cognitive decline, breathing a bit of new life into the amyloid hypothesis [1]. Trials of drugs designed to remove tau, the abnormal protein in neurofibrillary tangles, have all failed so far [2]. The development costs to design, test, produce, and conduct clinical trials on new drug candidates are enormous, costing hundreds of millions if not billions of dollars.

A parallel effort is under way to find out if some drugs already in use for other disorders might have a benefit in Alzheimer's disease. These are almost all inexpensive generic drugs, so the pharmaceutical industry is not interested in pursuing these leads. One drug company buried its own study that showed a small but significant decrease in the prevalence of Alzheimer's in patients taking the company's drug for rheumatoid arthritis [3]. The drug was nearing the end of its patent protection, so the company probably felt that there was no financial incentive to conduct the studies necessary to get FDA approval to market the drug for Alzheimer's. In fairness, the benefit was modest at best and might not have held up after a rigorous, prospective phase 3 trial.

Funding for these repurposing studies has mostly come from government and institutional grants for feasibility studies, and from nonprofit foundations such as the Alzheimer's Association. According to a recent open-access review paper, in February 2020 there were 53 dementia-related clinical trials underway involving 58 medications previously approved by the FDA for other indications [4]. Most of these old drugs (78%) were tested for possible disease-modifying activity, and the rest were tested for relief of symptoms associated with Alzheimer's including confusion, anxiety, depression, psychosis, and seizures. These drugs included agents normally used to treat cancer, cardiovascular problems, psychiatric or neurologic problems, inflammation, and diabetes. No breakthroughs have emerged from these trials yet and many are still on going. But two recent studies suggest that some of these drugs may be effective in certain subsets of Alzheimer's disease.

Levetiracetam (Keppra) is a commonly used drug in the treatment of several types of epileptic seizures, and it is generally well tolerated. A little over 20% of people with Alzheimer's have clinical seizures, most commonly complex partial seizures involving a change in behavior or confusion without overt jerking of the limbs or signs of a generalized seizure. However, up to 50% of people with Alzheimer's have subclinical seizures, abnormal electroencephalograms (EEG) showing a pattern of epileptic changes but with no overt clinical signs of a seizure. A recent study published in *JAMA Neurology* looked at the effects of a small dose of levetiracetam on several cognitive tests [5]. Tests of executive function showed improvement but only in those subjects who had abnormal EEGs with evidence of electrical seizure activity. In other words, levetiracetam may be able to improve some cognitive problems in Alzheimer's patients, but only in those for whom the cognitive impairment is associated with subclinical seizures.

Another paper published in *Nature Aging* used a clever technique to screen existing drugs for the ability to flip a switch in the transcription of the *APOE-4* gene in cell lines derived from *APOE-4* transgenic mice and *APOE-4* positive humans [6]. The most effective drug at flipping this *APOE-4* transcription switch was bumetanide (Bumex), a diuretic commonly used in older patients with severe edema and/or heart failure. In the *APOE-4* transgenic mice, beta-amyloid in the brain was markedly reduced after treatment with bumetanide. Also, the level of brain excitability returned to normal after exposure to bumetanide. An accessible discussion of this complicated paper can be found in *Alzforum* [7].

In order to see if these laboratory effects of bumetanide might have real-world value in preventing Alzheimer's, two large medical-record databases of patients over 65 were searched, one in California and one in New York. Compared to age and sex matched controls, the patients taking bumetanide in the California group were 35% less likely to have Alzheimer's. In the New York group, the effect was even stronger. The patients taking the drug were 65% less likely to have Alzheimer's than the controls. Further studies will be needed to confirm these results. A prospective clinical trial is planned to start next year.

What these two new studies have in common is that each drug seems to work only in a subset of people with Alzheimer's. The cognitive benefit of levetiracetam is found only in patients with seizure activity on their EEGs. Any benefit from bumetanide in slowing or preventing Alzheimer's will likely be found only in those who carry the *APOE-4* gene.

References

1   van Dyck CH, Swanson CJ, Aisen P, *et al*. Lecanemab in early Alzheimer's disease. *N Engl J Med* 2023; 388: 9–21. https://doi.org/10.1056/NEJMoa2212948.

2   Imbimbo BP, Balducci C, Ippati S, Watling M. Initial failures of anti-tau antibodies in Alzheimer's disease are reminiscent of the amyloid-β story. *Neural Regen Res* 2023; 18: 117–118. https://doi.org/10.4103/1673-5374 .340409. PMID: 35799522; PMCID: PMC9241406 (open access).

3   Rowland C. Pfizer had clues its blockbuster drug could prevent Alzheimer's. Why didn't it tell the world? *The Washington Post* 2019 (June 4). www.washingtonpost.com/ business/economy/pfizer-had-clues-its-blockbuster-drug-could-prevent-alzheimers-why-didnt-it-tell-the-world/2019/ 06/04/9092e08a-7a61-11e9-8bb7-0fc796cf2ec0_story.html (open access).

4   Bauzon J, Lee G, Cummings J. Repurposed agents in the Alzheimer's disease drug development pipeline. *Alz Res Therapy* 2020; 12: 98. https://doi.org/10.1186/s13195-020-00662-x (open access).

5   Vossel K, Ranasinghe KG, Beagle AJ, *et al*. Effect of levetiracetam on cognition in patients with Alzheimer disease with and without epileptiform activity: A randomized clinical trial. *JAMA Neurol* 2021; 78: 1345–1354. https://doi .org/10.1001/jamaneurol.2021.3310 (open access).

6   Taubes A, Nova P, Zalocusky KA, *et al*. Experimental and real-world evidence supporting the computational repurposing of bumetanide for *APOE4*-related Alzheimer's disease. *Nature Aging* 2021; 1: 932–947. https://doi.org/10.1038/s43587-021-00122-7.

7   Burke CW. Can an old diuretic drug disarm APOE4, prevent Alzheimer's? *Alzforum* 2021 (Oct 15). www .alzforum.org/news/research-news/can-old-diuretic-drug-disarm-apoe4-prevent-alzheimers (open access).

34 WRITING WHILE IMPAIRED

Two years ago, in February 2021, I began writing a blog that expanded on my book, *A Tattoo on my Brain: A Neurologist's Personal Battle against Alzheimer's Disease*. Some of the regular readers of that blog may have noticed that I have not posted for a while. I aimed at writing something every week. Sometimes I missed a week, but by the beginning of 2023, I was stuck for nearly month. The truth is I have been having a lot of trouble thinking of anything interesting to write. I literally sit staring at a blank screen on my computer, unable to start writing. After several weeks of frustration, it dawned on me that I have writer's block. That certainly is not surprising. Problems with verbal memory are often one of the first and sometimes, the very first sign of Alzheimer's disease. Trouble remembering words, mixing up words, and misspelling words are all issues that are becoming more common for me. Last week, while walking my dog Jack in a neighborhood we hadn't been to for a while, I tried and failed to come up with the name of the street we were on. I stopped walking and tried to remember the names of other streets in the neighborhood, and I couldn't think of any of them, including the name of the street I live on. I had no trouble knowing how the streets were connected and how to get from there to home, but I just couldn't think of the names of the streets. It was disturbing, but I suspected my memory for street names would return, and it did within a few minutes.

My experience with writer's block over the last few months inspired me to look into how professional writers have coped with the onset of dementia. Thomas DiBaggio, *Losing My Mind: An Intimate Look at Life with Alzheimer's* (2002), and Greg O'Brien, *On Pluto: Inside the Mind of Alzheimer's* (2018), are two examples of journalists who wrote eloquently about their own battles with Alzheimer's disease. Both of them have been inspirations for me in my attempts to express what it is like to live with dementia. But, what about writers who don't yet have a diagnosis of Alzheimer's or dementia? Retrospectively, can one find clues in their writings that might predict the incipient onset of dementia?

The writings of Iris Murdoch may be the perfect source to address this question. She was adamantly opposed to any editorial changes to her books. She wrote them all by hand, and what she sent to the publisher was what was printed. Thus, any changes in her writing-style over time were preserved. She wrote 27 novels between 1954 and 1995, and she was one of England's most celebrated writers. She was awarded the Booker prize for *The Sea, The Sea* in 1978 and, in 1987, she was named Dame Commander of the British Empire. According to a case report published in *Brain* in 2005, her final book, *Jackson's Dilemma*, published in 1995:

> ... was received 'respectfully' but without enthusiasm, and I.M. would later reveal that she had been dogged by an intense and distressing 'writer's block' while working on it. A year earlier she had become uncharacteristically inarticulate while taking part in an unscripted question-and-answer session about her work at a conference, and diary entries from 1993 are noted by her biographer as being reduced to heart-rending simplicity [1].

By the fall of 1997, she had clear signs of cognitive decline. A Mini-Mental State Exam (MMSE) score was 20/30 consistent with mild dementia. Six months later, the MMSE score had declined to 10/30, severe dementia. Extensive cognitive testing and an MRI scan were consistent with a diagnosis of

Alzheimer's dementia, and this was confirmed at autopsy after her death due to Alzheimer's dementia in February 1999, at age 79.

The fascinating paper in *Brain* goes on to report a retrospective, automated, textual analysis comparing three of her novels. *Under the Net* (1954) was her first published novel. *The Sea, The Sea* (1974) was written at the height of her literary career. And, *Jackson's Dilemma* (1995) was her final novel. The analysis showed evidence of a restricted vocabulary in the final book compared to the first two. Among the various technical findings, there was a greater rate of repetition of words in the final book and a greater rate of introduction of new words in the first two. In *Jackson's Dilemma*, she struggled to come up with words.

This should be no surprise. I can relate completely. I have a lot of trouble finding the word I want. It is a real problem whenever I am speaking. Writing seems to be a bit easier because I can look at the words I have already written, and the context helps me find the word I want next. Even though I am still in the mild stage of Alzheimer's dementia, any richness of vocabulary I might have had before is gone. I have to keep it simple. But that's OK. Look what Iris Murdoch could do writing *Jackson's Dilemma* while her Alzheimer's disease was probably at the stage mine is now. Good for her!

References

1   Garrard P, Maloney LM, Hodges JR, Patterson K. The effects of very early Alzheimer's disease on the characteristics of writing by a renowned author. *Brain* 2005; 128: 250–260. https://doi.org/10.1093/brain/awh341 (open access).

35 SPREADING THE WORD

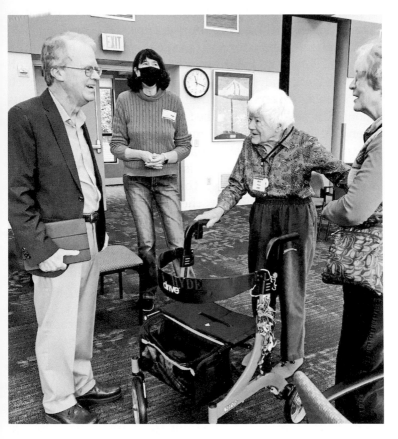

Photo by Lois Seed

My maternal grandfather and namesake, Daniel Martin, was a Presbyterian minister. Although I don't share his religious beliefs, I sometimes feel a bit like an itinerant preacher must feel, spreading lessons I have learned as a neurologist who now has Alzheimer's dementia. So far, I have spoken on at least 40 occasions for interviews on radio, TV, newspapers, magazines, and podcasts from around the world, from Dubai to New Zealand. I have also spoken to medical students, graduate students, other physicians, and Alzheimer's support groups.

Recently, I was honored to speak at a retirement community just down the hill from where I used to teach neurology residents and see patients in clinic at Oregon Health and Science University. I admit having been a little nervous about this talk. Over the last six months or so there has been a decline in my verbal memory, making it hard to stay on track during conversations. Reluctantly, I wrote out a script, but when the time came, I relaxed and went off script without too much embarrassment. When I couldn't remember the names of the Lawrence Livermore and Lawrence Berkeley National Laboratories (I had my PET scans done at the Lawrence Berkeley Laboratory), several members of the audience helped me find the words. I read two essays to the group. One called "Physician Heal Thyself" was published in the March 2023 issue of *Alzheimer's TODAY*, the official magazine of the Alzheimer's Foundation of America. I have reproduced it as Chapter 2 of this book. The other essay, "Living in the Moment with Alzheimer's," was originally written to be the last chapter of this book.

I was also a little nervous about this talk because the film crew for the documentary film based on *A Tattoo on my Brain* came to the event. It turned out to be fine. The audience didn't seem to mind a bit, even though they had to sign permission forms for the filming. They seemed to think it was all pretty interesting and fun. At one point, I went off

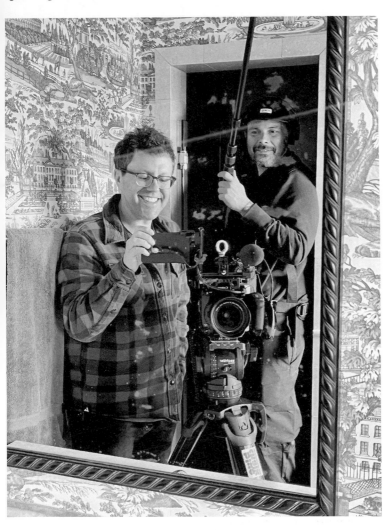

Rob and Jim filming me taking my daily pills.

script while talking about the film project, relating how the film crew had been in and around our house for three days in April 2022, and how they had gone out of their way to be as unobtrusive as possible. I mentioned how Jim, the sound-man, had been in our shower while Rob had been filming me taking my daily pills. I peered out into the audience looking for Jim and couldn't see him. I said something like "where is the soundman?" I immediately saw a number of pointing fingers and heard people calling out "he's in the closet." I had to chuckle.

36 SAYING GOODBYE
TO *LIZZIE G*

I have loved boats almost all of my life. When I was a small boy, my father and my great-uncle Fred taught me how to row and sail in a small dinghy. I was in awe of Uncle Fred for a number of reasons including his service in the US Navy in both World War I and World War II. My family never owned a boat during my life, but my father and I would occasionally sail the 26 miles to Catalina Island off the southern California coast with friends of his. Later, I spent several summers with my mother's cousin, Dick Stewart and his family, on their small island near Sidney, B.C. Cousin Dick was a lifelong boat lover and sailor. I remember when he sailed from Newport Beach in southern California all the way to Japan, while in his 70s. He returned along the coast of Russia and across the Aleutian Islands. He owned a variety of interesting power and sailboats over the years. I think my favorite may have been a tugboat that was built in 1906 with steam power and later converted to a diesel-powered pleasure craft named Point Hope. This may have been my inspiration 15 years ago when I bought a 25 ft mini-tugboat that I named *Lizzie G* after my mother, Elizabeth Gibbs. Honestly, my mother was not a fan of boats, but my father loved them, and I caught the bug from him.

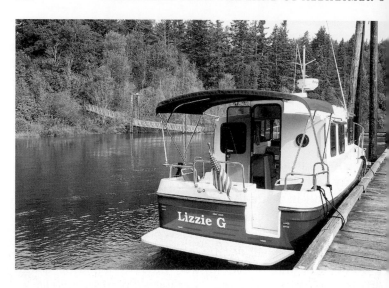

Over the last 15 years, I have explored the Columbia River west as far as the river's mouth at Astoria, 95 miles away from Portland and east, as far as the Bonneville Dam, about 37 miles away. I've also taken her up the Willamette River through downtown Portland as far as the dam at Oregon City. Lately, as my Alzheimer's disease has slowly progressed, it has become increasingly difficult to safely operate and maintain my beloved *Lizzie G*. So, with real sadness and a sense of loss, I have put her up for sale.

In the fall of 2022, my friend John Harland and I took *Lizzie G* for one more trip to Beacon Rock. September had been hotter than usual, and we struggled a bit hiking to the top in the heat. As always, the view from the top, 850 ft above the river was spectacular. What was striking this time was the shallowness of the river after an early snow melt and several months without rain.

Later, as we sat in the cockpit watching the setting sun light up the hills around us and sipping a beer, a solo canoer pulled up next to us at the dock. John Kraft is a young man who has been canoeing by himself from St.

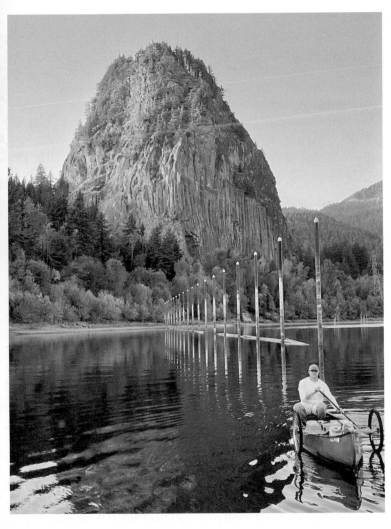

John Kraft in his canoe with Beacon Rock in the background. The bicycle wheels are used for portaging around dams. (A black and white version of this figure will appear in some formats. For the color version, refer to the plate section.)

Louis, Missouri to Astoria, Oregon, following the nearly 2,000-mile route of the Lewis and Clark expedition of 1804–1806.

The next morning, John Harland and I took a tranquil 1½ mile walk with no elevation gain through fields and woods originally belonging to the farm next to Beacon Rock State Park. The owners of the farm donated their land to the state of Washington, and it has made a wonderful addition to the state park. When we returned to the *Lizzie G*, John the canoe guy had left, still about six days out from his goal in Astoria. About a half hour after we left the dock, we encountered him again, paddling down river with the current.

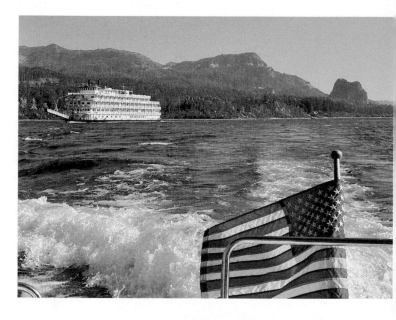

Soon, we picked up our final escort on *Lizzie G's* last trip, a sternwheeler taking tourists up and down the Columbia River. I had never seen it before except when it was docked in Portland, but as it passed us it seemed to be paying a fitting tribute to my fine little boat.

37 AMYLOID AND TAU PET SCANS OF MY BRAIN

In 2015 and again in 2018, I traveled to San Francisco to be a volunteer in a study of a then experimental PET scan for abnormal tau protein in the brain using a radioactive ligand called $[^{18}F]$-AV1451. This radioactive ligand binds with high affinity to insoluble, paired-helical filaments of hyperphosphorylated tau, the principal component of neurofibrillary tangles. Although my three-year follow up scans were delayed by the Covid-19 pandemic, I returned with Lois in September 2022 for a third set of studies spread over two days. What made this visit different, other than having to wear masks throughout the visit, was the presence of the film crew that is making a documentary film based on my first book, *A Tattoo on my Brain: A Neurologist's Personal Battle against Alzheimer's Disease.*

The first day was spent at the Sandler Neurosciences Center on the University of California San Francisco (UCSF) Mission Bay campus. I had several hours of cognitive testing, a comprehensive neurological exam, blood tests, and a high-resolution MRI scan of my brain to determine the amount of progressive loss of brain tissue. Lois was interviewed by psychologists for her take on my cognitive issues. The film team documented almost the entire day. Dr. Gil Rabinovici, the principal investigator for the study, and the entire team at the Sandler Neuroscience Center were amazingly accommodating and supportive of the film project. It was an exhausting day, but I think it was worth it.

The next day, Lois and I and the film team headed across the San Francisco Bay to the PET scan site at Lawrence Berkeley National Laboratory, building 55. The project director there, Dr. William Jagust, and the lab staff were very gracious in accommodating the filming. The scanning room at this site is connected by a pneumatic tube to a cyclotron two buildings away where the radioactive tracers are assembled. The beta-amyloid PET scan was performed using $[^{11}C]$-PiB (Pittsburg Compound B). As the radioactive carbon-11 (^{11}C) decays to boron-11, positrons are released and are detected by the scanner creating an image. This was the first successful ligand for amyloid PET scanning, and it still has features that make it an excellent choice, such as low off-target binding. The downside is that the radioactivity of ^{11}C decays with a half-life of only 20 minutes. After five half-lives, or 100 minutes, there is no longer any detectable radioactivity. It is currently used only as a research tool as it requires an onsite cyclotron and a tightly coordinated injection minutes after assembly. For me, the experience of the ^{11}C-PiB scan entailed lying on my back in a machine that is essentially a highly modified CT scanner. A standard CT scan is first performed creating black and white images of my brain. The radioactive ligand then arrives from the cyclotron through a pneumatic tube with a woosh and thunk, just as in the department stores when I was a small boy. At the precise, pre-determined moment following assembly, the radioactive ligand is injected into a catheter in my arm with no discomfort. Then, I lie still for 90 minutes while positron detectors create images based on the location of radiation in my brain. These colorful images are superimposed onto the black and white CT images of my brain. I don't begin to understand how this really works, but for me it was not hard at all. I actually slept through most of it. The film crew was there taking shots of me from all directions and recording the pneumatic arrival of the ligand.

The tau PET scan followed after the amyloid scan and was somewhat anti-climactic as it takes only 30 minutes of scanning. The [^{18}F]-AV1451 tracer has a half-life of 110 minutes so it is much easier to handle. In fact, a version of [^{18}F]-AV1451 has been FDA approved and is now marketed as Flortaucipir with offsite assembly. My tau PET scan used the onsite-assembled [^{18}F]-AV1451.

Both the amyloid and tau PET scans require computerized post-processing to create the color-coded images we are familiar with. So, it was several weeks before I could see the finished scans. Let's look at the amyloid PET first and compare it to the two previous amyloid PET scans done in 2015 and 2018.

In 2015, there was a moderate amount of amyloid in the cortical regions of my brain, especially in the prefrontal and frontal lobes. At this time, I had mild, subjective feelings of cognitive impairment, but my objective cognitive testing

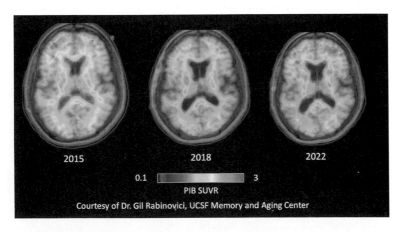

These are amyloid PET scans of my brain in 2015, 2018, and 2022. Beta-amyloid shows up as yellow, orange, and red depending on the amount in that area. These are horizontal slices through my brain at a level just above the eyes. (A black and white version of this figure will appear in some formats. For the color version, refer to the plate section.)

was still normal. In 2016, I enrolled in a clinical trial of the anti-amyloid monoclonal antibody, aducanumab. For 18 months, I received monthly infusions of what turned out to be a placebo. In September 2017, I entered an open label extension study during which I received the active drug every month. Just before Christmas, I developed the most severe headache of my life, combined with severe confusion and extremely high blood pressure, requiring ICU care. I have discussed this severe episode of amyloid-related imaging abnormalities (ARIA) in Chapter 13 of my book *A Tattoo on my Brain* [1] and in a case report published in *Alzheimer's & Dementia* [2]. As shown in the MRI below, I had evidence of swelling in multiple areas throughout my brain.

It took about six months to fully recover from the ARIA episode. I returned to UCSF for another set of PET scans about nine months after the ARIA event. As seen in the amyloid PET scan above, in 2018, there was actually less amyloid seen in my brain. As we now know, aducanumab and similar drugs are actually quite effective at removing amyloid from the brain, and after just four doses, there was

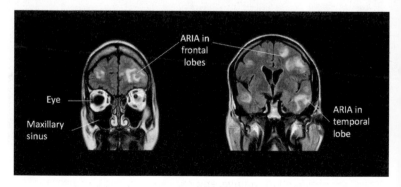

This is an MRI scan from 2017 showing multiple areas of brain swelling called amyloid-related imaging abnormalities (ARIA). These are vertical slices through my brain. Adapted from an image in A Tattoo on my Brain: A Neurologist's Personal Battle against Alzheimer's Disease.

less in my brain. However, that benefit was not sustained. As the last amyloid PET scan above shows, by the fall of 2022, the amyloid had returned and progressed.

What about tau? Recall that tau is the abnormal protein found in the neurofibrillary tangles of Alzheimer's disease. It can first be detected a few years before the onset of cognitive impairment. As shown in my tau PET scans below, in 2015, when I had very mild cognitive impairment, there was just the beginning of tau deposition in the anterior temporal lobes, especially on the left. In 2018 and again in 2022, the tau had spread on both sides. This is the part of the brain where short term memory is consolidated into long term memory, so it is not surprising that my cognitive testing shows worsening of verbal memory. But, the rest of my brain still looks pretty good, both on the tau PET scans and in the cognitive tests.

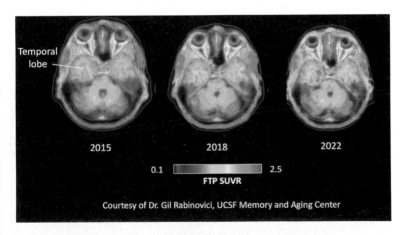

Courtesy of Dr. Gil Rabinovici, UCSF Memory and Aging Center

These are tau PET scans of my brain at the level of the eyes and anterior temporal lobes. Yellow, orange, and red represent increasing concentrations of tau. The intense red in the eyes is off-target labeling that appears in normal people as well. (A black and white version of this figure will appear in some formats. For the color version, refer to the plate section.)

I am very encouraged by these studies. My Alzheimer's disease is progressing very slowly. Damage to my brain has been limited mostly to the temporal lobes and olfactory centers. Extensive cognitive testing now puts me in the border zone between mild cognitive impairment and mild dementia. I am still largely independent in my activities of daily living, although I now rely on Lois to handle the family finances. I can still read and write, although my reading speed has decreased, and I sometimes struggle to come up with something interesting to write. I don't know exactly why my Alzheimer's is progressing so slowly. Perhaps I have some unidentified genetic factor that counteracts the effects of my two *APOE-4* alleles. Perhaps I have enough cognitive reserve to keep my brain functioning for a while longer. Perhaps the lifestyle changes I adopted are making a difference. Maybe the four doses of aducanumab did something useful, although I think it is unlikely. Whatever the cause, life is still good, and I intend to keep doing everything I can to keep it that way.

References

1   Gibbs DM, Barker TH. *A Tattoo on my Brain: A Neurologist's Personal Battle against Alzheimer's Disease* (second edition). Cambridge: Cambridge University Press, 2023, pp. 93–97.
2   VandeVrede L, Gibbs DM, Koestler M, et al. Symptomatic amyloid-related imaging abnormalities in an APOE ε4/ε4 patient treated with aducanumab. *Alzheimers Dement* 2020; 12: e12101. https:doi.org/10.1002/dad2.12101 (open access).

38 RUNNING ON A FIELD OF DREAMS

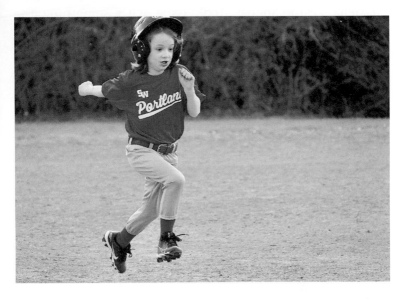

My 7-year-old grandson James airborne last spring during his very first little league baseball game.

I love baseball. I was never any good at it myself. I have memories of watching in shame as the ball rolled between my legs in left field. Later, when the pitchers started throwing breaking balls, I could never tell what was coming to me as a batter, probably because I wouldn't wear my glasses. In my last game playing baseball in eighth grade, I was hit in the face by a fast ball that I mistook for a curve. I kept waiting for the trajectory of the ball to change, but alas it never did.

No, I wasn't any good as a player, but I loved to watch the game. Growing up in Southern California, I rooted for the Los Angeles Dodgers. Those were the days of the great pitchers, Don Drysdale and Sandy Koufax, and the base-stealing shortstop, Maury Wills. My baseball glove was the "Don Drysdale Signature" model. The Dodgers' archrivals were, and still are, the San Francisco Giants. I remember watching a game on TV when San Francisco pitcher, Juan Marichal, came to bat, took issue with something the Dodger catcher John Roseboro said, and then turned around and hit Roseboro on the head with his bat. A melee ensued. But, as evil as the Giants seemed to a young Dodgers fan, I couldn't help but admire their center fielder, Willie Mays, one of the most spectacular players of all time. It seemed that no fly ball would ever make it past him unless it was hit out of the park.

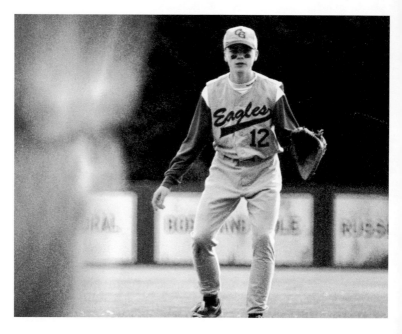

My son Adam playing in the infield during high school.

My son Adam and daughter Susannah played baseball and softball competitively all the way through high school. They were both much better at the game than I ever was. Lois and I spent many afternoons watching them play each spring, often in the Oregon rain. I adjusted my work schedule as much as possible, and I don't think I missed many home games.

Now, James is excited about the coming season. The kids get to pitch this year, and he is hoping to be a pitcher. Maddie, his younger sister, is gearing up for T-ball, so we will have a double schedule of games to watch this season. I suspect Adam will be involved in coaching both teams. Watching my son pass along his love of baseball to his children is about as good as it gets.

39 LIVING IN THE MOMENT WITH ALZHEIMER'S

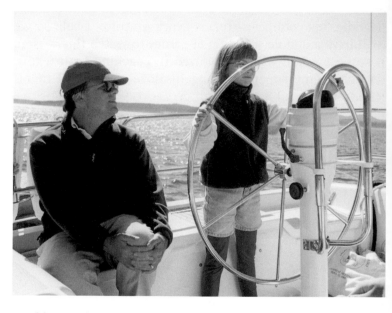

Teaching my daughter Susannah how to sail in 1999.

When we are young, the timeline of our lives stretches from our earliest memories to our expectations for the future. As the cognitive impairment of Alzheimer's disease progresses, that timeline begins to constrict. Perhaps surprisingly, the first memories that start to go are the most recent – where did I put that (fill in the blank)? The consolidation of new memories in the hippocampus is impaired, while our ability to remember events from the distant past is relatively well preserved in a variety of cortical regions of the brain. As time goes on and the amyloid plaques and neurofibrillary tangles spread throughout the brain, the distant memories start to fade. The memories most likely to endure are those that are associated with strong emotional content, but eventually even those start to disappear. At the same time, our abilities to look into the future and make plans become impaired as damage spreads to the prefrontal cortex. Eventually, in the late stages of Alzheimer's, we are left with life in the present – no past and no future. I'm not there yet, but I can sense the shrinking timeline of memories from the past and plans for the future. For those of us on the Alzheimer's journey, it is really important to embrace the moment and not dwell on the frustration of trying to remember the past and plan for the future. Others can help us retrieve old memories. Calendars, lists, and post-it notes will help us minimize the chaos of the future. But happiness and peace come from focusing on the moment, whether it is hugging a grandchild, writing in a journal, working in the garden, or listening to great music. As Horace put it over two thousand years ago, *carpe diem quam minimum credula postero* – seize the day and don't worry about tomorrow.

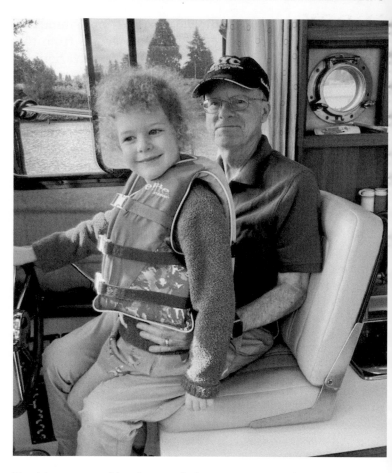

Teaching my granddaughter Emily how to steer a straight course in 2022.

INDEX